TAKING CONTROL WHEN YOU'RE NAKED

a Guide for the Savvy Health Care Consumer

David C. Fisher, Ph.D.

To Uncle Sherry –
Love, Dave

NPI

Northwest Publishing Inc.
5949 South 350 West
Salt Lake City, Utah 84107
801-266-5900

NPI

LC/CB 10293

This book is not intended as a substitute for diagnosis and treatment by trained health care professionals. The reader should always seek the opinions of the most appropriate practitioner for treatment of his or her particular health concerns.

The author and the publisher disclaim all liability and responsibility resulting from the use of the procedures, sources of information, and help discussed and/or recommended in this book.

ISBN 1-56901-087-0

First printing 1994

Printed In the United States of America

To Anita, Laura, and Alissa.

Acknowledgments

This book would not have been possible without the help of people with a wide range of training, skills, and experience. Health care professionals who made contributions or suggestions include Katherine Gray, Ph.D., John Newcome, M.D., Julia Rice, M.A. L.I.C.S.W., and Mark Schuler, Ph.D..

Christine Brunkhorst, M.A. and Anita Fisher assisted by making editorial comments that undoubtedly made this a more readable manuscript.

Contents

Preface

This book was written to help you get the best possible treatment in today's health care system. It was inspired by many people who have improved the quality of their care by becoming knowledgeable, assertive consumers, even at times when they felt frightened and vulnerable. These people have studied their problems and have actively directed their treatments. They've felt free to question advice and work with a variety of health care professionals. It is this attentiveness, along with the willingness to be treated by different caregivers that is everyone's best guarantee of receiving high quality health care.

A few words about language. The term "patient" is generally not used in this book. This is because the word has often been used to describe people who were unable to control their own treatment. In other words, to many a patient is someone who passively relies on another person, usually a doctor, to make decisions. In its place I have used "consumer" and "customer" because these terms emphasize the skills people now often have to learn to receive competent treatment. Similarly, the term "doctor" is usually avoided. Unfortunately today it often suggests a person who is given control over someone else. As you will find out, I strongly discourage these types of relationships. Instead, the terms "caregiver," "practitioner," and "professional" are used because they don't carry some of the unwanted connotations of the word "doctor." They also emphasize that there are now many nonphysician health professionals who also provide highly skilled care.

In the following pages, I will illustrate actual experiences people have had being treated for various illnesses. Of course, information that could reveal true identities has been altered.

—David Fisher

Part 1

Working the System

CHAPTER 1

The New World of Health Care

"Toto, I've a feeling we're not in Kansas any more."

– Dorothy (**The Wizard of OZ,** ***1939)***

High Priced Success

Lately, we have witnessed a dramatic improvement in the ability of health care practitioners to keep their customers healthy. This success is reflected, in part, by the increase in life expectancy from 45 to 75 years in less than a century. Our sophisticated medical technology deserves a good share of the credit for this achievement. Less than one hundred years ago children often had rickets, and many people died from now curable diseases like smallpox and syphilis. There was no penicillin to fight infections, X-ray equipment to look at broken bones, or even aspirin for headaches. Hospital wards may have had thirty or more ill people in the same room. In those days, people were also given more harmful treatments or frequently exposed to others with contagious diseases. In fact, at the turn of the century going to a hospital was probably more often a curse than a cure. Now, once undreamed of procedures such as organ transplants, successful cancer treatments, and kidney dialysis are commonplace in a modern medical center. Sanitation is excellent and hospitals offer more privacy. In an effort to increase profits, many hospitals even entice consumers with gourmet meals, cable TV, and plush carpeting.

These advances have come at a price. Consider, for example, a recently developed machine called a Magnetic Resonance Imager. This equipment, referred to as a "MRI," allows images to be taken that are similar to X-rays. It makes it possible to diagnose accurately a wide range of illnesses with much greater ease and precision than ever before. Each MRI machine, however, costs millions of dollars. To make a profit, most hospitals charge consumers from $1,000 to $1,300 for each MRI test. While the family physician of years past may have been able to carry most of his or her supplies in a little black bag, today's physician must frequently rely on such incredibly expensive equipment to meet present day standards for high quality medical care.

In most areas of the United States the physician who makes house calls and then stays for a bite to eat is a thing of the past. Medicine is now big business. Consider the salaries earned by physicians. The average physician now makes over $150,000 each year with some topping $500,000. It is also common for a surgeon to charge from $3000 to $6000 for a single operation taking three or four hours. Although it would be easy to lay most of the blame for the high cost of health care on physicians, they are not the only practitioners who charge high prices. Many others, including psychologists, nurses, speech therapists, and acupuncturists, demand over $100 an hour for their services. Hospitals also contribute, sometimes charging $2.50 for a single Aspirin tablet and $400 a day for a hospital room. Not surprisingly, you may find that the price of being in the hospital can easily reach $10,000 a week.

Cut Rate Care

In the past when consumers did not have medical insurance they could often pay for their treatments with their savings. In the 1950s, when many of us were born, every day in a maternity ward cost the typical family a little less than two days' earnings. With today's hospital stays now costing much more, most households rely on insurance to pay for health care. Not only is this insurance expensive, but there are a staggering variety of insurance options available. Today's consumer can often choose to have traditional insurance or to be covered by new institutions such as "preferred provider organizations" and "health maintenance organizations." Sometimes they can even be covered by specialized insurance plans designed for one corporation's employees. Each type of coverage has different rules regarding what treatments will be covered. To further complicate things, many health plans usually pay only a percentage of the bill. Sometimes insurers won't even cover any costs if they decide the consumers are not getting the care they need. Regrettably, ill people may not know about such limitations until after they become ill.

Knowing about the coverage provided by a health insurance plan is especially important for today's consumers. Some health insurance plans, in an effort to reduce costs, offer poorer health care coverage. These plans may make it difficult for you to visit a specialist, receive second or third opinions, or see the same caregiver each time you visit their clinic.

Unfortunately, recent economic conditions make it impossible for many families to afford more expensive, but often higher quality, health insurance. How many households today would be able to pay an extra $200 each month for an insurance plan that won't hassle them when they need to be treated quickly or require long term care in a nursing home? The reality is that consumers need to find the best health insurance they can afford, even if it is lacking in some respects. For many, this search results in poor quality care. Either a good insurance plan is not available in their community, or they don't know enough about medical insurance to make a wise choice. Fortunate and informed consumers however, are able to find excellent care at reasonable prices.

Perhaps those worst off are those who have no health insurance at all. One study (Hadley, Steinberg, & Feder, 1991) showed that people with no insurance were up to three times as likely to die as people with private insurance. The uninsured were also much less likely to receive high cost treatments such as knee replacements or heart bypass surgery.

Technology

Understandably, many people have also felt overwhelmed by today's sophisticated health care technology. They wonder how they could ever hope to learn the uses of a MRI or know the intricacies of fields with unfamiliar names like hematology, rheumatology, dietetics, or cardiology. One unfortunate result of this is that many consumers don't even attempt to educate themselves about their medical conditions. Instead, they believe that the care they are receiving is beyond their ability to understand. In other words many sick people are not becoming informed consumers; they are not learning about their illnesses, questioning decisions made for them by others, or consulting another practitioner who they think would give them better care. It is ironic that few of these people would be so unwilling to question their own automobile mechanic whom they suspect is charging them for poor car maintenance.

In part, this problem occurs because it is often more difficult for people to do research on their own medical conditions than it is for them to get second opinions on whether their cars need new tail pipes. When ill, consumers can be at quite a disadvantage. They may not have the physical or emotional strength to investigate health problems, health insurance plans may restrict their ability to get other opinions, and there may not be enough time to study an illness.

Having an illness should not mean giving up trying to understand the decisions made on your behalf. Fortunately, there are now many ways for people to learn about their medical problems. Librarians can use computers to search hundreds of journals for articles about your illness in a matter of minutes. Book stores contain a tremendous amount of information from a range of specialists. There are also many more health care providers today than in years past for you to contact. It takes a knowledgeable person to take advantage of these opportunities and learn how to make the best use of health care services.

When You're Sick for a Long Time

Another consequence of today's health care technology is that people often have to deal with the discomfort of long term treatment. While the person with cancer many years ago may have died, today's consumer may pay the price of living by enduring treatments that cause such side effects as hair loss, nausea, and vomiting. Diagnosis and treatment may involve frightening or painful medical tests, all of which are essential for survival. Although he or she lives longer, this person may have to cope with many unfamiliar problems. These new difficulties are often poorly understood by the friends and family that are normally turned to for help and emotional support.

Thus, in some ways medical technology seems to make it even more difficult to live with the cancer. Enduring these procedures often means learning new relaxation skills or teaching family members how to be more helpful. Today there are many opportunities to learn such techniques. Psychologists, psychiatric social workers, chaplains, physicians, and others can teach people to handle their illnesses. With their help, the knowledgeable consumer can take advantage of new and innovative treatments that a range of professionals offer.

Minorities

Minority groups can face special difficulties when trying to find good health care. For example, many are often forced to go to low-cost or public hospitals, some of which offer poor quality care and probably have higher death rates than private hospitals used by whites (Hartz et al., 1989). Most of the public hospitals in New York, for example, provide no routine mammogram screening. Even worse, a third of the people diagnosed with breast cancer in those public facilities receive no follow-up care. The death rates from breast cancer in these hospitals are almost three times the national average (Beck et al. 1990).

Another problem is that in many parts of the country black mothers are much more likely than white mothers to have babies that die shortly after birth. Some people (Hamburger, 1989) have suggested that this has been caused by black mothers' reluctance to take advantage of available prenatal care. Black women in Minnesota have often stated that they were not comfortable going to physicians who were usually white (Nyberg, in Hamburger, 1989). Others have not been able to go to medical appointments because of transportation problems, ambivalence about their pregnancies, personal or family problems, and difficulty making child care arrangements (Lia-Hoagberg, Rode, Bellfield, & Skovholt, 1988). Thus, many low-income women didn't receive the care they needed. Also, the state often did not tell minority women about the health care services available. It is striking that this problem occurred in Minnesota, the state that was the first to guarantee medical care for women and children regardless of their ability to pay. It is also a state where health service is a huge industry, employing more people and making larger profits even than agriculture.

Better Training and the Guilds

Caregivers from nurses to speech therapists now receive much more training than they did years ago. This results in an overall improvement in the quality of health care. Another advancement has been the formation of many professional "guilds." These have been created partly to insure that the public continues to receive competent care from well-trained practitioners. Each of these organizations helps regulate the practice of a particular health care specialty. For example, physicians have formed the American Medical Association (AMA). This is a multi-million dollar organization that, among other things, decides what training physicians should receive, publishes books and professional journals, educates the public, and directs medical research.

One of the most important functions of the AMA is to protect the public from unqualified persons attempting to practice medicine. To do this, the AMA has successfully lobbied for regulations that prevented persons without adequate medical training from becoming licensed physicians. Similarly, other professional guilds have also worked to give their own practitioners exclusive legal rights to provide consumers with specific types of health care. As a result, only dentists may extract teeth, only psychologists may do psychological testing, and only nurses may attend to many of a hospitalized person's needs. These laws are similar to those that require the person you hire to fix your sink to be a trained plumber. In each case the members of a guild have convinced lawmakers that they are the only ones who should be allowed to provide certain services.

Professional Rivalries

Although guilds have probably improved the overall quality of health care, they have also caused some problems for consumers. These have primarily stemmed from the efforts of certain guilds to prevent members of other organizations from treating consumers. This is often done with claims that practitioners from other guilds are not competent to diagnose or treat a particular problem. The American Medical Association, for example, has fought many times to make it necessary for people to receive referrals from physicians before insurance plans will pay for treatment by practitioners without medical degrees. They argue that only a physician is qualified to diagnose and treat many disorders. Naturally, other caregivers have opposed such restraints claiming that they restricted consumers' freedom to choose their own practitioner. With billions of dollars at stake, these turf battles are often vicious and costly.

The American Psychiatric Association (part of the AMA) and the American Psychological Association, are two groups that have often battled with each other. Each of these organizations represents practitioners with a specialized type of training. Members of the American Psychiatric Association are physicians, called "psychiatrists," who specialize in treating mental illness. Presently, they are the only practitioners trained to prescribe medication for mental disorders. Because these practitioners began their education by studying medicine, their training usually emphasizes biological causes of mental disorders. For example, if a psychiatrist was treating a depressed person that professional might have a tendency to look for medical problems that could be causing the person's emotional distress. Diagnosis and treatment might consist of an interview, medication, and sometimes medical tests or counseling.

In contrast, psychologists, who are usually members of the American Psychological Association, receive training that generally emphasizes the contribution of behavior and environment to mental illness. Consequently, a psychologist will often spend more time discovering what it is about the person's environment or activities that makes him or her depressed. While treatment might include referral to a psychiatrist for medication, the psychologist is more likely to help the person feel better by behaving differently.[1]

Both the psychologist and the psychiatrist lend important perspectives to mental health care. The talents of each may be essential to help someone with emotional difficulties. In ideal situations these two specialists work together. A depressed person may, for example, first visit a psychiatrist who will evaluate the causes of the depression. After this evaluation the psychiatrist may decide that the person would benefit from antidepressant medication. The psychiatrist may also notice that the person's life is in turmoil because of marriage or job difficulties, physical illness, and so forth. At this point the physician may refer the person to a psychologist for counseling to help manage stress. Together then, the psychologist and the psychiatrist help, both with medication and by teaching the person to deal with problems more effectively. The scientific research shows that this "teamwork" is the most effective way to treat many emotional problems.

Rather than work together like this, psychologists, psychiatrists, and other caregivers sometimes choose to compete with each other, often at consumers' expense. Here, a psychologist may not tell the depressed person that a psychiatrist could prescribe a medicine that might help. A psychiatrist, in turn, may recommend medication but not help the person cope with stress. The same problems exist between members of other competing guilds. Chiropractors might not refer their customers to surgeons when needed just as social workers can refuse to send people to psychiatrists for necessary medication.

Because of competition between different guilds, some specialists make misleading statements to the public about the causes of health problems. More often than not these claims are meant to

1 — These descriptions are admittedly stereotyped and do not describe all persons practicing in these fields. There are many psychiatrists who take more of an interest in helping people with counseling just as there are psychologists who specialize in biological causes of mental illness. Perhaps the ideal is to have a mental health practitioner who is well versed in the interplay between both behavioral and physical causes of emotional distress. However, as with many areas of health care, practitioners cannot learn all there is to know about several fields and, consequently, often restrict training to a specialized area.

prevent the consumer from looking for help from a practitioner within another specialty. For example, psychiatrists sometimes say that emotional problems are caused by "chemical imbalances in the brain." While often true, this statement is occasionally used to prevent treatment by other specialists who do not have medical degrees. After all, if the problem is only medical (a "chemical imbalance") a psychiatrist (who, is a physician) would be the only person qualified to treat the disorder. The contributions of, say, occupational or marital stress are dismissed. This may discourage the consumer from finding other perhaps more appropriate care.

Let's look at some other ways this competition can affect your treatment. Imagine that you have been going to your family physician for several years because of back pain. During this time the physician has treated you with medication to reduce muscle spasms and has assured you that there was nothing more that could have been done. While this may be true, the physician might not know about the therapies that other practitioners offer. Many times this lack of knowledge is caused by caregivers' tendencies to stay away from members of competing guilds. In other words, they don't hobnob enough with professionals who offer alternate treatments. The result is that they may not know enough to refer you to someone who might be able to give you genuine relief.

Your practitioner also might be worried about losing your business by referring you to someone else. This concern is a surprise to many consumers. They naively believe that practitioners won't let financial worries stop them from sending customers to more helpful caregivers. Like most people though, health care practitioners are interested in making money. Unfortunately this may prevent a few of them from sending you elsewhere for care when you need it most.

There is also the problem of ego. Some caregivers see themselves as great healers, able to cure any malady that comes through their door. Of course it doesn't work this way in reality. Too often they feel powerless when they can't help a desperately ill person. They may see it as a personal failure to send you to somebody else and be embarrassed by the limitations of their own skills.

With these problems in mind, it is clear that today's street-wise consumers are usually the ones most wary of the practitioners who try to discourage them from visiting competitors. Instead, they seek out the practitioner who is more open to considering help from those who have different areas of expertise.

A New Look at Illness

Before the 1950s the medical model was generally the most accepted way of viewing illness. In this model people had diseases that were largely unrelated to social or emotional factors. Headaches, for example, were described primarily as a medical problem best treated with medications. Other, non-medical, causes of headaches such as stress were de-emphasized, if not ignored. Input from professionals other than a physician may not even have been considered.

In the late 1950s the World Health Organization advocated a more comprehensive model of health care. In this new system, psychological and social aspects of illness are considered in addition to the physiological. For our headache sufferer, this means a much more comprehensive treatment plan. Not only may this person have medicine prescribed by a physician, but treatment might include visits to such specialists as psychologists and social workers. When working with the person, these professionals might first help find stresses that trigger the headaches. With some work it may become clear that the pain gets worse during times of financial difficulty. The psychologist may then teach the person muscle relaxation skills while the social worker could assist in finding a better job. The combination of medical, social, and psychological treatments therefore may be used to help the person more than medication alone. This new, more comprehensive, model of illness has placed more emphasis on caregivers who help people both psychologically and socially. Physicians now work closely with professionals in these fields to deliver, as a team, the best treatment possible today.

The experienced health care consumer, working with professionals from many areas of expertise, soon learns that treatment may depend largely upon the specialties of the practitioners. We know that the physician, for example, might look at headaches as uncontrollable spasms of blood vessels in the brain. The social worker could likely see them as reactions to a difficult occupation; and, the psychologist may look at them as the result of excess muscle tension. Probably for similar reasons one woman (Prior, 1987) received conflicting advice on whether or not to have a mastectomy for her breast cancer. It is clear that her caregivers' conflicting recommendations may have been greatly influenced by their different areas of expertise.

> *When the lump did turn out to be malignant the surgeon came and held my hand and told me that he thought I should have a mastectomy.... The radio therapist did arrive at the end of the afternoon and having examined me said that so far as he was concerned I could keep my breast and have radiotherapy... The next morning he returned to warn me that the surgeon would be coming back to try to persuade me to have the operation... Approaches to breast cancer should not vary so much from one hospital to another, nor should treatment be dependent on the opinion of one surgeon. It should not be, as one doctor put it, "a kind of lucky dip."*

In a similar way, a person with cancer might be told by a physician that an upset stomach is a side effect of cancer fighting medication. Because of this, the physician may change the anti cancer drugs to reduce the likelihood of similar symptoms occurring in the future. While this may help, another physician specializing in disorders of the digestive system may be asked for a second opinion. This second physician could discover that the person has a stomach ulcer that makes an upset stomach especially likely. Consequently, more medication and dietary changes may be recommended to help treat the ulcer.

Finally, the psychologist and the dietician might notice that the person becomes much sicker just before eating certain types of food. In other words, "food aversions" have developed where the sight or even the thought of certain foods makes the person ill. This is very much like what happens when someone's mouth waters at the sight of Thanksgiving dinner. In both cases the body has learned to react (with either nausea or salivation) to the sight of food. While the dietician may recommend dietary changes, the psychologist may help the person gradually be exposed to the food in a way that will slowly reduce the discomfort. Again, the purpose for having so many specialists is to be able to look at illness from different perspectives. This often leads to different diagnoses and treatments, each of which may help customers with their problems.

A health care system that relies on the services of different types of caregivers is particularly important now that physicians rarely make house calls. Many years ago, when physicians often saw people at home, they were able to see a more complete picture of the person's life (Reiser, 1978). For example, they could talk with the person's spouse to learn if medication was taken on time. They might notice if screaming children prevented the person from sleeping or see if the person with poor balance had to walk up a tall staircase. Today's office-bound physician is at a great disadvantage when it comes to knowing about everything that may have an impact on the customers' health (Reiser, 1978). Consequently, physicians now rely on other practitioners to learn about the many aspects of people's lives that directly affect their well-being.

Freedom Of Choice

Historically, physicians have been the only health care practitioners to be paid without question by insurance companies. In the past before a practitioner from another specialty could be paid that caregiver had to jump through two hoops. First, it was necessary to show that the customer had originally been referred to that practitioner by a physician. Second, the caregiver needed to treat the person according to the physician's instructions. These requirements meant that consumers went to physicians first, and then the physicians decided if they could go to another practitioner in a different specialty area. Furthermore, the physicians usually chose the treatment the ill person received even after they were sent to the other caregiver.

This custom often denied the consumer the freedom to work with practitioners from many specialties. In other words, they were stuck with the caregivers the physicians chose. In the past twenty years or so, however, lawmakers have given consumers much more power in choosing their own health care providers. Because of this, health insurance companies will now usually pay for your treatment by chiropractors, psychiatric social workers, psychologists, and many others without requiring you to receive a referral from a physician first.

Because of these changes, the physician, who was once given almost all of the power, now has less ability to dictate treatment decisions. The power that the physician lost has been given to the consumer. This gives you much more ability to control your own health care. You can now play an active role in choosing the practitioner who you believe will best treat your illness. It may be a physician, a psychologist, a nurse, a nurse-midwife, or someone from many other professions, depending on your assessment of your own needs.

This new control makes it essential that you be able to make smart decisions about your own health care. To do this you may need to learn about many things, including the causes of disease, different treatments offered by a variety of practitioners, and health insurance plans. You may have to become assertive with health care providers and ask appropriate questions. You also might want to learn about new methods to reduce your anxiety or physical discomfort. This book is designed to help you take initiative and responsibility for your own care in these and other ways. It is intended to help you make wise choices and stay well in today's rapidly changing health care system.

CHAPTER 2

What to Look For When Hiring a Caregiver

"He must really be a wonderful wizard to live in a city like that."

—Dorothy (**The Wizard Of OZ,** ***1939)***

Getting a Referral

In recent years consumers have become incredibly sophisticated in judging the quality of all sorts of goods and services. Witness, for example, the popularity of consumer magazines that scrutinize everything from toothpaste to automobiles. These are read by millions to make sure that their tires will last, their roofs will not leak, and their microwave ovens will heat evenly. The readers of these magazines might use many other tactics to insure the best value for their dollar. These include comparing the value of items at different stores or asking the advice of a friend before making a purchase.

We spend a lifetime learning about buying products. Think, for example, about the first time you purchased an expensive item such as a car. You may have asked the salesperson questions about the car's repair record, cost, and safety. You may have pretended that you weren't interested so the salesperson would be tempted to quote you a lower price. You could have asked about other similar cars on display in the showroom. These tactics helped you learn about automobiles and enabled you to pay the lowest price possible. Also, they made you a more sophisticated consumer for the next time you needed to buy an automobile. Years later, if you were pleased with the car, you may have bought another. If it was a lemon though, you probably shopped someplace else.

Health care is another product that consumers learn about largely by asking questions. Before they receive proper care though they may try many disappointing treatments or visit many caregivers. Only with experience, knowledge, and some luck do most consumers eventually find the help they need.

Your selections of caregivers will be some of the most

important decisions you will make during your illness. These will be the people who you may rely on to help you make crucial health care decisions. While the well-trained practitioner can be invaluable in your treatment, the wrong professional could easily jeopardize your recovery. Certainly then, it is in your best interests to know enough about various health professionals to make the most informed choice about which ones you will hire.

Consumers often look for new health care practitioners when they move to a different area, or, perhaps more frequently, when they have a health problem that their present caregiver can't treat. If your current practitioner isn't trained to help you with an illness that professional should recommend that you see someone who has had experience working with that problem. It reflects very positively on your original caregiver if you are referred to another practitioner. This is because caregivers, who are often in intense competition with each other, sometimes only reluctantly send customers elsewhere. McClure (1985) complained that when this happens professionals may call other practitioners on the telephone to ask for free treatment advice rather than send the customer to another office for more competent care. In other words, one caregiver might call another and say: "I've got a difficult one here and I don't know what to do. How would you handle this problem?" It would often benefit the customer to actually be treated by the other caregiver and not just rely on the advice that professional gave over the telephone.

If you are fortunate enough to have a caregiver who will send you elsewhere when necessary, that referral advice can be quite valuable. This is because your present caregiver, like many seasoned professionals, probably can quickly identify the most skilled practitioners in your area. Your current professional likely has had the benefit of watching many other practitioners work. For example, your caregiver might remember the best surgeons when recalling the outcomes of their past operations. It may have taken years to get this knowledge. As a consumer of health care, you probably don't have the luxury of spending a great deal of time locating the most competent surgeon. Therefore, you might do well to seriously consider advice from such people with more experience and knowledge than yourself.

While this advice may be valuable, it should not be followed blindly. One reason to think about these suggestions is even your trusted practitioner may be basing the referral on things other than the next caregiver's competence. For example, it is common for practitioners to work together in "groups." The members of these groups often share office space and secretarial services. Some may send you to a caregiver in their own group even if that person is not the most qualified person in your community to treat your illness. One reason for this is sometimes financial. Your original practitioner may benefit by referring you to someone else in his or her professional group because your business helps pay both of their office expenses.

There are, however, advantages to working with more than one professional in the same group. With the busy schedules practitioners often endure, sharing office space may help them communicate quickly with each other. This may be especially important if your treatment is complicated and requires the services of many people. In these circumstances it may be crucial for all of them to have your health care history available on a moment's notice.

Professionals working in the same group also may know a lot about the other members' skills and weaknesses. Ideally, if one person is especially good at working with a particular disease that practitioner is likely to get more customers with that illness from other members of the group. Similarly, if that caregiver isn't very good at working with a problem the other professionals will probably steer consumers with that illness away from the caregiver. This is another advantage to working with members of the same professional group. Each may be able to send you to a colleague whose skills and limitations are well known.

In certain situations it is especially likely that you will be treated by more than one provider from the same group. When a woman is ready to deliver a baby her physician may be home in bed. If this happens one of the other members of that physician's group will usually be summoned to assist in the delivery. This allows the woman's original physician to keep a more predictable schedule and get some sleep. Thus, when deciding to work with a caregiver who practices in a group, it may be important to interview the other professionals in that practice. This will give you the chance to see if you are comfortable with them and judge the quality of care they are likely to provide.

Another reason people are sometimes sent to a specific professional is because that caregiver happens to be next on a referral list. Hospitals, in particular, generally keep lists of practitioners in a variety of specialty areas. Names on these lists may be given to consumers who call in on the telephone or are newly admitted to the hospital. These lists generally only contain the names of caregivers who work in that hospital. They usually do not include the names of other, possibly more experienced, practitioners who work in other hospitals in the same geographic area. They also usually do not have information about a practitioner's professional degrees, years of experience, and so forth. Thus, when a hospital gives you the name of a practitioner, it is not necessarily the most skilled person practicing in your location.

These lists also might contain just the names of physicians. Other qualified caregivers such as licensed clinical social workers or registered nurses may not be included. Their names are often left out because physicians, who have a tremendous amount of power in hospitals, usually want customers to be sent to them first.

Quite often people will use telephone referral services that are designed to give referrals to a specific kind of health care provider. These numbers are often found in the yellow pages. Such referral lines are usually set up by professional guilds that want to advertise their members' services. Guild members are often put on these lists after paying a fee and informing the referral service of the types of people they are most qualified to treat. For example, a psychologist might tell a service that he or she would prefer to receive referrals from callers who are having difficulty with, say, marital relationships. The referral line would then refer callers with marital conflict to that psychologist.

Such services probably save consumers time in locating professionals with particular specialties. The majority of caregivers receiving the referrals from these lines are also likely to be members in good standing of a particular guild. Since most guilds have at least some minimal standards for membership (education, licensure, years experience, etc.), the consumer can often have some confidence in the credentials of the professionals recommended by these referral services. As with the hospital referral lines discussed earlier though, these services may not suggest you see professionals in other guilds. Again, the consumer is forced to be self-educated about the services offered by caregivers with a variety of specialty areas.

Another reason to examine referrals results from professionals' general reluctance to criticize other caregivers. I remember one woman who was diagnosed with a brain tumor. A friend of hers gave her the name of a well-known surgeon who was very experienced in performing the delicate surgery she needed. His qualifications, attested to by a wall of diplomas and certificates, were exceptional. With these assurances she thought he was probably one of the best surgeons in the area. So, she decided to schedule surgery.

She then told her social worker and dietician of this decision. These caregivers knew that her surgeon had a generally poor reputation in the professional community. They also knew that he had bought some expensive laser surgery equipment and made a practice of using it on most of his customers. With this equipment he could make incisions without a knife blade. Instead, he operated using a concentrated beam of light that easily burned through tissue. This equipment is often helpful because it is precise and causes little bleeding. This particular laser equipment, however, could overheat brain tissue when used in this surgery. In this operation, such heat would have likely damaged healthy brain cells surrounding her tumor.

The other professionals also knew that the surgeon had removed too much brain tissue during many of his previous operations. Some people suffered unnecessary problems such as difficulty swallowing, understanding speech, and moving limbs. They were particularly worried because the surgeon also told his new customer that he may have to remove part of her brainstem. The brainstem is a part of the brain that controls such necessary functions as heart rate, breathing, and the swallowing reflex. If a piece of her brainstem were removed, it would be likely that she would also needlessly suffer problems similar to those of his earlier customers.

After hearing of her surgeon's plans, the social worker and the dietician discussed between themselves the advice they would give the woman. Their decision was to emphasize that she get a second opinion from another physician. They did not tell her that her present surgeon's plan was probably quite dangerous. To do so would have been considered professionally inappropriate. They were not physicians trained in the surgery and were not qualified to dispute his recommendations.

Luckily, the woman listened to the concerns of those urging her to get another opinion. When she consulted another surgeon, she was told that there were much safer and equally effective surgical techniques available. These methods did not require removal of a portion of the brainstem or present the risk of damaging healthy tissue with too much heat.

The advice from the woman's nonphysician health care providers was appropriate. They shifted the responsibility of making an informed choice back to her, where it belonged. They also weren't qualified to give a medical opinion even though they had good reason to believe that the planned medical treatment was inappropriate.

Finding a Caregiver Near You

Your choice of health provider will largely depend on your knowledge of the professionals in your community. Perhaps you live in an area that offers a wide variety of services. Often the best selection of health professionals is in larger metropolitan areas where there is much demand for health care. If you look through the telephone book of a major city you will probably be able to find a smorgasbord of professionals with many different types of training. You can locate everything from a geneticist to a dietician without much trouble. If this variety of care is available in your community, your job of finding someone to help you with your problems will be much easier.

Or perhaps you live in an area that offers few choices. Tragically, many smaller towns or isolated rural communities have no practitioner qualified to perform such essential services as delivering babies and setting broken bones. In other areas there may be only one or two health care practitioners. Unfortunately, people may unfairly expect them to provide health care for a wide range of problems that they are not competent to treat. This is particularly dangerous because these caregivers often feel compelled to deliver services that they have not been trained to perform. We have all heard stories about veterinarians who have set broken bones in humans. More commonly though, we might see things like general physicians asked to do mental health counseling or chiropractors called upon to treat stomach ailments. These professionals may feel the need to "do something" to help their neighbors any way they can. And after all, by receiving their services their customers might be better off than if they received no help at all. Problems sometimes occur when customers leave their offices with the mistaken impression that they have received high-quality care. Unfortunately, the only way they may actually find competent health care may be to make a trip to a larger city.

When selecting a caregiver, you may also want to keep in mind that there is generally more opportunity for urban professionals to receive continuing education. Continuing education usually consists of classes to increase the practitioners' knowledge and/or skill. For example, classes for nurses might emphasize the latest methods of administering medication for pain control or for helping people reduce anxiety. The urban professional can often take these courses without traveling more than five or ten miles from home. On the other hand, caregivers in rural areas may have to travel hundreds of miles to benefit from this same training.

Specialists

Most consumers are unfamiliar with the training and services caregivers in a modern medical center provide. "What is the difference between a psychologist and a psychiatrist?" and "What kind of training does a movement therapist have?" are the kinds of questions many consumers ask. Below are descriptions of the training and skills of some of these practitioners.

Certified therapeutic recreational specialist

Certified therapeutic recreational specialists perform a variety of jobs that center on helping people engage in more satisfying and productive leisure activities. The many benefits of this therapy include improved physical abilities, increased involvement in the community, more effective stress management skills, and higher self-confidence.

While most of these therapists have bachelor's degrees in therapeutic recreation, some have earned masters or even doctoral degrees. During school they have been given hands-on training working with people. All students receiving certification in this field must also pass a national written exam.

Chiropractor

Chiropractors believe that many illnesses are caused by problems with the nervous system. They view these problems as triggering symptoms such as headache, bedwetting, chronic pain, and even difficulties with the immune system. One of their most common treatments involves moving vertebrae that are believed to be causing problems with the nervous system because they are out of alignment. This may be done by forcing, or "manipulating" them into proper alignment in the spinal column. This spinal manipulation is perhaps the most traditional treatment performed by chiropractors. It is, in fact, the primary treatment offered by some chiropractors who went to school many years ago. More recently, however, schools of chiropractic have emphasized courses in areas such as nutrition, exercise, and even acupuncture. While some chiropractors (often referred to as "straights" by their peers) still primarily treat people by spinal manipulation, others are now treating people with a variety of these newer and sometimes controversial techniques.

Chiropractors have a long and occasionally contentious history with other caregivers. Because of this, their relationship with other practitioners deserves special comment. Until very recently, even the American Medical Association did not allow physicians to refer people to chiropractors. It was not until the chiropractors filed a lawsuit against the AMA that this policy changed. Basically, the chiropractors' claim was that the AMA policy of preventing referrals to chiropractors illegally discouraged competition between professionals. The supreme court agreed. And, because of this decision, physicians are now permitted to send customers to chiropractors. Occasionally, chiropractors now share office space with physicians and even practice in hospitals under their direct supervision.

Training for chiropractors varies somewhat from state to state. Generally though, they first complete at least two years of undergraduate university classes, taking science courses such as biology, chemistry, and physics. Next, they enter a college of chiropractic for about four years. In this school they take classes and also actually treat people. During chiropractic college, students are required to pass national board exams. Shortly thereafter they complete tests given by their particular state professional organization before they become licensed to practice chiropractic.

Dance/movement therapist

Dance/movement therapists work with movement and dance as a form of psychotherapy. They are skilled in helping people pay attention to nonverbal communication and expression. They work in places as diverse as hospitals, mental health clinics, and even prisons. Often dance/movement therapy is not the only treatment people receive, but instead is used along with a variety of other treatment approaches.

Generally, after finishing four year bachelor's and two year master's degrees, dance/movement therapists are granted D.T.R. ("dance therapy registered") or A.D.T.R. ("academy of dance therapists registered") status. Persons with the A.D.T.R. degree have met additional requirements allowing them to teach and supervise other dance/movement therapists and engage in private practice. Their courses include study in observation and research skills, psychology, choreography, improvisation, and classes on psychological problems. In school they are also required to be supervised while treating a variety of people.

Dietician (registered)

Dieticians work in a variety of settings: hospitals, research laboratories, day care centers, schools, and even in corporations that develop new food products. Your work with dieticians is most likely to center on helping you learn what foods will be healthier for you to eat. Your dietician should consider your individual needs when planning your meals.

A registered dietician first completes a four-year undergraduate bachelor's degree, often in nutrition, dietetics, or food systems management. Some students go further in school and earn either master's or doctoral degrees. Training also involves supervised hands-on work in the field of dietetics. After completing this training, the student is required to pass a national exam before being allowed to call him or herself a "registered dietician."

Nurse

Nurses perform a staggering variety of health care services ranging from care of the person with heart disease to counseling the mentally ill. Not only can they be found in hospitals, but some have their own clinics staffed entirely by nurses.

Nurses generally must complete twelve months to four years of nursing school after high school or college. There now is a trend toward training in four-year nursing schools instead of in the shorter programs. All nursing programs must be approved by a Board of Nursing in that particular state. After completing nursing school the student must pass a written examination to become either a "licensed practical nurse" (LPN) or a "registered nurse" (RN). Generally an RN will have completed more years of school than a LPN. In addition, LPN's are sometimes restricted from performing duties such as passing medication, engaging in private practice, or accepting supervisory positions in hospitals.

Nurse-midwife (certified)

A certified nurse-midwife's skills include providing regular gynecological services such as pap smears and breast exams.

Also, they can educate you during pregnancy, help in the delivery, and offer advice on the care of the newborn. Each nurse-midwife works closely with a physician in case problems arise.

Certified nurse-midwives first receive their training in nursing school where they become registered nurses. Next, they attend accredited schools in nurse-midwifery for one and one-half to two more years. Then they earn either master's degrees or certificates in nurse-midwifery. Finally, they have to pass a national written examination given by the American College of Nurse-Midwives. Do not confuse a certified nurse-midwife with a with a lay midwife. Lay midwives are usually nonprofessionals who do not necessarily have the same training as certified nurse-midwifes.

Pharmacist

In the hospital or drugstore, the pharmacist does much more than count pills. They are often seen by other caregivers as the best source for information on how certain drugs may react with other medications, affect the human body, or be effective in the treatment of disease. Pharmacists also serve as a safeguard against the improper use of medications by other hospital personnel. Although you may never see them in the hospital, they might come to your room or review your medical chart in order to make recommendations for your care.

Pharmacists first complete a five-year undergraduate bachelor's degree in pharmacy. Some continue for two more years to receive either master's or doctoral degrees. Of those who have received doctoral degrees, some complete one to three years additional training in a residency or fellowship program. Pharmacists must pass both a written national exam and a state exam before they are licensed to practice pharmacy.

Physician

Historically a physician's role has been to be "in charge" of health care. This has meant that physicians have been the only professionals to order medical tests, supervise other caregivers, and to be paid directly by insurance companies. Although physicians are still often the most commonly used health care professional, their role is changing as caregivers with other degrees are being better trained and are taking more active leadership positions. For example, other professionals such as nurses and social workers are now often paid directly by insurance companies for providing consumers with health care services. Psychologists can admit people into some hospitals and take full responsibility for their care. No physician may need to be involved, much less take charge, in many of the treatments provided by these practitioners.

To be licensed with an M.D. (medical doctor) degree, a person must first graduate from college and then from medical school. It usually takes eight years to complete this training. Next, the new M.D. must finish a one-year "internship," an experience that provides actual experience treating illness. Students also need to pass at least one written national examination before becoming licensed. Although they can legally practice medicine at this time, most go on to two to nine more years of "residency" training to learn a specialty area. Further written national exams may be required, depending on the area in which the M.D. chooses to specialize.

Another type of physician is an osteopath. They provide many of the same services as M.D.'s, such as perform physicals, prescribe medication, and do surgery. These practitioners, comprising about 5% of the physicians in the U.S.A. (American Osteopathic Association, undated — A) have somewhat different training than those with M.D. degrees. Their degree is called a D.O. or Doctor of Osteopathy. In order to become an osteopathic physician, students must first complete at least three years of college courses after high school. Although graduation is not required, almost all earn bachelor's degrees before entering a college of osteopathic medicine. Students attend colleges of osteopathic medicine for four years, and take science courses such as anatomy, pharmacology, and biochemistry. In addition, during this training they study fields such as surgery, radiology, preventive medicine, and pediatrics. After graduation, they complete a one-year internship during which they refine their skills by treating people with a variety of illnesses. Although they are qualified to practice medicine after their internship, many go on to training in a residency program which takes from two to six years to complete. This experience makes it possible for them to later practice in hospitals, which generally require this more extensive practical training. During their residency, students further specialize in a specific area such as anesthesia, family medicine, or surgery. The students also must pass national tests at the end of their second year of osteopathic school, before graduation. In addition, they must sit for whatever licensing exams their particular state requires. This licensure is required in all states.

Although their training is remarkably similar, there are differences between D.O.'s and M.D.'s. First, osteopathic physicians often say that they believe in a more holistic model of health care than do M.D.'s. They state that they place more emphasis on how different organ systems affect each other. For example, they believe that many problems with internal organs are caused by the body's poor ability to tolerate standing erect. They think that standing upright subjects the body to the downward force of gravity, something that the spinal column and internal organs are often not able to tolerate. They believe that one result of this is excess strain on the muscles and bones. When the muscles contract because of physical or emotional stress, these problems may worsen. An osteopathic physician's treatment for such problems might include physical manipulation to loosen the muscles and joints. They believe that this relaxation eventually may help internal organs heal (American Osteopathic Association, undated — B). M.D.'s, on the other hand, generally do not offer these treatments which are designed to counteract the effects of gravity.

Also, some osteopathic physicians provide a somewhat broader range of services than M.D.'s. For example, it's not uncommon for one osteopathic physician to treat children, perform gynecological exams, and deliver babies. By offering so many services, they function in many ways like family practice physicians who also treat people regardless of age. There are also many hospitals that are staffed primarily by osteopathic physicians who often provide essentially the same services as people with M.D. degrees.

Specializations of M.D.'s and D.O.'s include such intimidating names as otolaryngology, gastroenterology, endocrinology, and neonatology. Often, physicians will refer to themselves as "throat doctors" or "stomach doctors" and so forth to help people remember. While this may help, it is often not detailed enough information for you to be able to understand thoroughly their training or role in your care. To make things clear below is a list of a few physician specialty areas along with brief explanations of the problems each specialist treats.

Anesthesiologist

A specialist in the use of medications that block the sensations of pain and feeling, or result in the loss of consciousness. If you have surgery, an anesthesiologist would probably be the person who would "knock you out" before surgery and help you breathe during your operation.

Cardiologist

Diagnoses and treats problems of the heart and blood vessels.

Cardiovascular Surgeon

These practitioners perform surgery on the heart and the surrounding blood vessels.

Dermatologist

Diagnoses and treats skin problems.

Endocrinologist

Diagnoses and treats diseases of organs that release hormones in the body. Consumers often work with endocrinologists when they have diabetes, thyroid problems, or growth abnormalities.

Family Practice Physician

Specializes in providing and coordinating medical care for family members, regardless of their age.

Gastroenterologist

Diagnoses and treats problems with the digestive system (the esophagus, stomach, intestines, colon, rectum, and anus).

General Practitioner

Much the same as family practice physicians. They specialize in providing care for a broad range of illnesses that do not require the services of another specialist. Often you may first visit a general practitioner who will be the first to diagnose your illness. If necessary, he or she will then refer you to another practitioner who specializes in treating that particular problem.

General Surgeon

Performs many "general" surgeries such as appendectomies, hernia repair, and gallbladder removal that do not require the services of a specialist in another area.

Gynecologist

Diagnoses and treats women's reproductive organs.

Hematologist

Specialist in the diagnosis and treatment of diseases involving the blood and bone marrow (the place where blood cells are manufactured).

Infectious Disease Specialist

Specialist in the diagnosis and treatment of diseases (spread by "microorganisms") that can spread from one person to another.

Internal Medicine Specialist

Sometimes called "internists," these practitioners most frequently treat diseases involving problems with the heart and blood vessels, the liver, the gastrointestinal tract, and the blood. They generally do not perform surgery.

Neonatologist

Diagnoses and treats disorders that occur within one month after birth.

Nephrologist

Diagnoses and treats disorders of the kidneys. These are the organs that filter blood and produce urine. People will often work with a nephrologist if they are on kidney dialysis or if they have diabetes and also have kidney damage.

Neurologist

Treats disorders of the nervous system (brain, spinal cord, and other nerves).

Obstetrician

Cares for pregnant women and delivers babies.

Occupational Medicine Specialist

Helps to prevent and treat illness and injury that occur at the work place or as the result of an occupation.

Oncologist

Diagnoses and treats cancer.

Ophthalmologist

A physician who diagnoses and treats diseases and other problems with the eye.

Don't confuse this physician with "optometrists" or "opticians." An "optometrist" examines eyes for problems and may prescribe eyeglasses. An "optician" makes eyeglasses as directed by an ophthalmologist or an optometrist. An optician, however, does not examine eyes or treat problems with vision.

Otolaryngologist

Performs surgery and treats disorders of the ear, nose and throat. Often referred to as an "E.N.T." physician.

Perinatologist

Diagnoses and treats the fetus just before birth and the infant during the first month of life.

Physical Medicine and Rehabilitation Specialist

Sometimes called "physiatrists." They specialize in the use of physical therapies such as exercise, electrical stimulation, mechanical braces, etc., for the treatment of the physically disabled.

Psychiatrist

Treats emotional problems. May use drug therapy, counseling, or other methods to treat mental illness.

Radiologist

Diagnoses and treats diseases with X-rays or similar means. These practitioners may be the ones to look at X-rays, interpret CT or MRI scan results, or direct the radiation therapy for a person with cancer.

Rheumatologist

Diagnoses and treats disorders in the joints and connective tissues such as tendons, ligaments, and the skin. Common illnesses they treat include arthritis, bursitis, and gout.

Physician's assistant

Duties are quite diverse and include taking case histories, assisting with emergencies in the absence of the physician, helping with laboratory tests and physical examinations, giving injections, and suggesting diagnoses and treatments. By relying on physician's assistants to perform many of these tasks, the costs of health care are usually reduced because the services of a physician are not necessary. This also allows the physician to spend time working with customers who have more complicated or urgent problems. The physician's assistant works under the supervision of a physician, who is responsible for the quality of care they provide. Many physicians' assistants work in rural areas, where other caregivers are often not available.

To become a physician's assistant, students usually complete at least two years of college along with some other work experience in the general field of health care. Then, they enter a physicians' assistant training program, typically for another two years. During this time they take classes in areas such as pharmacology, biochemistry, physiology and general medicine. After finishing school and successfully passing a national examination, the physician's assistant must pass another written examination every six years. This is necessary to maintain certification by the National Commission on Certification of Physician Assistants.

Psychologist

There are many specialty areas within psychology. In a

hospital, it is possible that you will work with professionals called "neuropsychologists." These caregivers are trained to find out if people have problems with such skills as concentration, reasoning, and memory. Quite frequently medical problems such as head injuries, brain tumors, heart difficulties, or certain medications will cause people to have these types of difficulties.

In the hospital you may also work with a psychologist specializing in areas referred to as "behavioral medicine" or "health care." These psychologists are experts in looking at the contribution of people's behavior to their physical condition. For example, these psychologists might understand how your stress leads to headaches, how your anxiety contributes to high blood pressure and overeating, or how you can reduce your pain through the use of muscle relaxation techniques.

In most states, after graduating from college, a psychologist is required to have a total of five years training in graduate school to receive a doctoral degree. This includes at least one year of "internship" working with people in hospitals, mental health centers, and other settings. Some psychologists go further and receive post-doctoral training in a specialty area. To become licensed, they usually then have to complete one or more years of supervised training treating customers. They also must pass national and local tests.

Registered occupational therapist

These professionals assist people who are unable to function normally because of aging, physical injury, emotional difficulties, or abnormal development when growing up. Using a number of techniques, they attempt to help people become more self-sufficient. These techniques include helping physically handicapped people use devices such as wheelchairs, specially modified spoons, clamps to hold pencils, or shoe horns. These caregivers may help the handicapped person exercise to improve strength or flexibility. They may also help people with memory difficulties or other problems learn to organize and carry out daily tasks.

The registered occupational therapist's credentials include a four-year college bachelor's degree, usually in occupational therapy, as well as six to nine months of supervised internship working with physically and emotionally handicapped people. In addition, others have completed two to four years of graduate school for masters or doctoral degrees in occupational therapy. They also must pass a national examination before being allowed to practice.

Social Worker

Social workers perform a broad range of services. Perhaps one of their most common activities is to help people locate or use community resources. This might include helping people get assistance from an appropriate food shelf, nursing home, or government organization. Also, social workers often do psychotherapy as well as participate in a variety of community services. These can range from planning community health projects to advocating for the homeless. They work in settings such as hospitals, private practice clinics, nursing homes, schools, and crisis intervention programs.

While training varies by state, all new social workers in the U.S. are required to have a four-year college bachelor's degree. If this degree is in the field of social work it is referred to as a "bachelor's of social work" (B.S.W.). This degree will generally will qualify social workers to be employed in entry-level positions in many hospitals, government agencies, and clinics. In order to be qualified to do private practice and directly charge consumers for their services, social workers are required to attend two more years of school to earn a "master's of social work" (M.S.W.) degree. Both the B.S.W. and M.S.W. degree programs include classes in human behavior, counseling and interview skills, helping people use government programs, and research methods. Both degrees also include supervised work helping actual clients. Most states require social workers to be licensed.

Speech-Language Therapist

If you are having difficulty speaking, listening, writing, or reading, you might work with a speech-language therapist. These communication problems have a variety of causes that include stroke or head injury, poor blood circulation, and slow or abnormal development as a child. Speech-language therapists help people improve such communication skills. Also, many speech-language therapists treat people who have trouble swallowing due to many of the same causes.

In some states, speech-language therapists are required to hold a Certificate of Clinical Competence in Speech-Language Pathology. To receive this certificate they must have a master's or doctoral degree and also have completed courses in fields such as science, math, and biology. In addition, they need to spend hundreds of hours observing the work of other speech-language therapists and treating language disorders themselves. Finally, they are required to pass a national written examination.

It is often very helpful if many of these professionals work in your area or hospital because each has unique skills. Consider how a team of these caregivers might help a person who is paralyzed in an automobile accident. The physician will probably first diagnose the physical injury to the person's back. The physician will then recommend surgery or other measures to stabilize the damaged spine. Soon after, a physical therapist may help the person to regain leg strength with exercises. Also, the psychologist or psychiatrist may diagnose or treat problems such as depression and anxiety, or provide education about sexuality. Occupational therapists may help the person relearn typing, driving, or eating skills or once again to perform many other daily activities essential to living a relatively normal life.

In this scenario, the caregivers may also suspect the injured person suffered brain damage during the accident. If this happens, a physician will probably recommend that a special X-ray, called a CT scan, be taken to look for physical changes in the brain. It is often the case, however, that these pictures will show a perfectly looking brain while, at the same time, the person may have severe difficulties remembering, for example, how to schedule appointments, even with the help of a calendar. The person might also go into a rage each time a minor frustration such as a traffic light is encountered. Each of these problems suggests that some brain damage occurred despite the normal CT scan.

Because of these problems, a neuropsychologist might perform testing to investigate the person's difficulties thinking. During this exam the psychologist will probably ask the person to work on many different problems. For example, he or she may do math, put together puzzles, define words, or draw pictures of simple designs. Each of these tasks measures skills in a different area. When a person has problems on one or more of these tests, the psychologist sometimes concludes that brain damage did occur. Thus, it may not be possible to diagnose a head injury from X-rays alone. The services of a number of professionals, looking at both medical tests and the person's behavior, are often needed to detect brain damage.

Each caregiver also might help rehabilitate the person once the brain injury has occurred. Speech problems could be corrected with the help of a speech-language therapist. A cognitive retraining specialist may help improve memory. Occupational therapists might show the person how to be better organized, and psychologists might teach the person to control anger. Again, a variety of specialists may make important contributions to the person's care.

One test of true professionals is to see if they try to look at illness in different ways, not just from within the constraints of their own training. In other words, these caregivers will recognize the limitations of their own knowledge and rely, as much as possible, on the unique perspectives that caregivers from other specialties may have. This is what makes a professional a scientist. They are open to input from others and do not insist that their model of illness is necessarily the correct one to follow. When your health care provider relies on other team members, each of whom can add something unique to your care, it is likely that he or she is one of these scientists. It is with that person that you will probably get the best care, and he or she is the one who deserves your trust.

Fortunately, you can usually spot the caregivers who insist their way is the only way. They are those who scoff at your ideas if they don't fit neatly into the treatment plan already devised. They may seldom work with a team of professionals, insisting that their input is not necessary. When you see such things happen, it may be a smart move for you to find another practitioner. Your present caregiver's narrow outlook is likely to make it difficult for you to work with the variety of professionals that you may need.

But What Are Their Qualifications?

You probably will want to ask your practitioners many questions about their training and qualifications. This is just like a job interview when an employer (you!) asks an applicant about education and past experience. While questioning a caregiver like this may have been quite a radical idea just a few years ago, today it is almost standard practice. In fact, asking appropriate questions about training and expertise often earns you the professional's respect and may encourage them to treat you as an intelligent consumer.

Many people are concerned that they will offend their caregivers if they ask about training and experience. Some of them even decide to avoid asking questions that may, in fact, be important. While this could help you to avoid bruising some egos, it could also result in your suffering at the hands of a less-than-skilled professional. A better solution might be to ask questions in a way that will get you the information you need with less chance of insulting your provider. Unfortunately, this may be difficult with a few professionals. The mere fact that you ask questions, no matter how respectfully, just plain irritates them. I've found that the best attitude for consumers is often to accept the fact that there is always the risk of this happening. To most people it seems a small price to pay to increase the chances of receiving better care.

Still, it's probably in your best interests to make your relationship with your caregiver as comfortable as possible. One study (cited in Cousins, 1983, pp. 163-164) looked at people with cancer who went against the advice of their physicians and took Laetrile, a drug that almost all physicians in the United States believed was not effective for the treatment of cancer. The purpose of the study was to find out what these people had in common. In other words, did they have a certain level of education, income, or ethnic background that made them more likely to go against their physicians' advice? The results of the study were surprising. The one thing that the people had in common was a poor relationship with their physicians.

One way to minimize the fallout from your questions and keep a better relationship with your caregiver is to speak with a nurse, secretary, or office worker before you make your first appointment. They often can give basic information about the provider's training and experience such as academic degrees, years experience, and so forth. This makes it possible for you to screen the caregiver over the telephone while maintaining your anonymity.

And remember, some people want to see their caregivers as heroes. Unfortunately, this may prevent them from looking more closely at credentials. One physician (Spooner, 1987) described a tendency for some people to need to feel that they are being "swept away" by someone who will cure all of their problems. These people may be the ones to describe their caregivers as "the best in the city" when their skills are actually mediocre. Spooner describes this phenomenon as a rather subtle form of regression. It is here where the consumer believes it's O.K. to turn all the responsibility for treatment over to a caregiver. This obviously can be a very dangerous way for the consumer to avoid having to take responsibility for his or her own care. It may be especially difficult for people to recognize this type of hero worship in themselves because it is such a subtle and often unconscious maneuver. Keep in mind then that your admiration for your caregiver should not stop you from asking about qualifications.

Another mistake is to measure a caregiver's medical competence from their bedside manner. This often happens to people who don't know how to judge a practitioner's skills by asking the right questions. One of the only things they can evaluate that professional by is their personality. Remember though that congeniality doesn't make a good surgeon. Nor does it make a good physical therapist, nurse, or pharmacist. The nicest and most caring practitioner in the world could still be incompetent when it comes to doing the job right.

As often occurs with consumers who mistakenly think their caregivers are "the best in the city" then, people who idolize practitioners because they are nice are also opening the door to trouble. Although a friendly caregiver is always desirable, most people place a higher priority on skill. They aren't paying for niceties, they are paying for quality health care.

Below is a list of questions that may be helpful for telephone screening or later when talking to your caregiver. Although this list covers some basic information that may be important to know, there will probably be other questions about your illness that you will want to ask.

1. How many people with my problem have you treated before?
2. (For physicians) Are you board certified to do this surgery or procedure? (Board certification means that they have met the requirements of a national board to practice a specialty of medicine. There are over twenty such specialties that include almost every area in medicine, including plastic surgery, dermatology, and pediatrics. The requirements of the national board usually include a certain amount of specialized training as well as the successful completion of a written test.)
3. How many of the people you have treated have recovered? How much better did they get?
4. Overall, what success rates do other professionals in your field have in treating this problem?
5. Are there other providers in this area who have treated more people with this problem than you have?
6. What academic degrees do you hold?
7. Are you licensed?
8. Have you written any articles on this illness?
9. Do you work with professionals from other specialties who might offer a different type of treatment for my problem?
10. Where do you work on different days of the week? (Many practitioners have several offices in different locations. Whenever you need to see them they always seem to be out of town at a distant clinic.)
11. Do you anticipate retiring or moving your practice to

another location in the near future?

12. From what university did you graduate?
13. At which hospital(s) do you treat people?
14. How difficult is it to arrange an appointment with you on short notice?
15. May I call you to ask a question over the telephone?
16. Does your office have:
    a. convenient parking
    b. wheelchair ramps
    c. easy and close access to public transportation?

It might be especially important for you to ask about board certification (see question number two) if you are planning to be treated in a physician's office instead of in a hospital. This is because physicians who have not been board certified are allowed to perform whatever treatment they have the nerve to do in the privacy of their own offices. For example, if they have only taken a weekend course in cosmetic surgery there is nothing that legally prevents them from giving you a facelift as long as they do it in their own offices. It's different, though, in most hospitals. In order for physicians to do certain types of treatment in hospitals, they often need to be board certified. This is because national organizations responsible for policing hospitals often require physicians to have this credential.

Be creative when asking questions and try to anticipate problems that could occur during your treatment. With technically difficult surgeries or rare health problems, it may be especially important to ask about experience. You may also want to get an idea of your provider's knowledge of other professionals' skills if you think you will need their help. Other consumers place a high priority on finding a professional who has the courage to say that they don't know an answer to a question. Rather than pretending to know all the answers, these professionals are more likely to be straightforward and to rely, when necessary, on help from practitioners with other types of training.

In some cases, you might ask to speak with a few of the caregiver's past customers to learn their impressions of the care they received. If you are working with a dentist, you may want to learn how closely that practitioner was able to match the color of a new crown to the other teeth. Or, you may want to see the handiwork of a plastic surgeon first hand before you decide to have your nose trimmed. Most practitioners will not give you the names of former customers, however, without their permission. And of course, there are some circumstances where releasing the names of former customers would be inappropriate. This would be the case, for example, with people treated for many mental health problems.

Sometimes when you ask about degrees, training, and other qualifications you will learn that your provider is still in school. She might be a student doing her "internship" or "residency." You are probably more likely to work with a number of these students if you are being treated in a university hospital. One sometimes annoying problem when working with students is that they may visit your room in small groups. Although some people enjoy the company of all the younger faces, others see their presence as a violation of privacy. If this is the case with you, you might request they visit you less frequently.

There may also be a tendency for these aspiring professionals to perform too many tests (Greenland, Mushlin, & Griner, 1979). These not only serve to satisfy their voracious curiosities, but also reduce the chances of them missing a problem that they might not have learned to recognize themselves. In other words, they may perform many different tests on you that a more experienced caregiver would not consider necessary.

Seeing one of these caregivers is a bit like getting a haircut at a barber college. You generally pay less (or nothing) for their services while taking a chance with their inexperience. These people usually have their work supervised, however, especially when it comes to important decisions. But, what they lack in experience is often made up in enthusiasm and openness. They may be eager to discuss your illness and give you more complete information than would other more seasoned providers.

Another thing that you may want to consider when you select a caregiver is the hospitals in which that person works. For example, many psychologists only treat people in one hospital. If that hospital has an especially bad reputation you might think twice about choosing that particular psychologist. The same is true of physicians, who generally are awarded "admitting privileges" to only a few hospitals in one area.

Finally, don't be afraid to ask how much a practitioner charges. Your caregiver may charge more than your insurance plan considers to be "reasonable and customary." If this is the case you may have to pay a large portion of the bill yourself. To avoid this try bargaining with your caregiver. Many professionals are willing to reduce their fees, especially for people who have financial problems.

Second Opinions

Many people avoid getting second opinions because they are concerned that their current caregivers will be offended. These are usually consumers who, for whatever reason, stick with a practitioner even though that person doesn't like to be questioned. If this is your situation, don't forget that you can have the second practitioner keep your visit a secret. This is common these days and the second practitioner is usually legally required to honor your privacy.

During your first visit to a practitioner's office you may want to make it clear just who you want informed about your condition. Many caregivers will assume that it's O.K. for them to tell your spouse or other relatives how you are doing when, in fact, you would prefer that all information comes from you.

Seeing someone else for a confidential second opinion has other advantages. First, if you are really worried about offending your original practitioner the second opinion will give you a chance to ask more direct questions. You won't have to worry about how this second caregiver feels because you may not see that person again anyway. You also don't have to worry about getting a reputation for being a "bad patient." This is because the second caregiver can't tell anyone about anything that you said.

Many people who seek second opinions go to caregivers who do not work with their original practitioners. This not only provides a better assurance of privacy but in many cases can result in a less biased second opinion. Sometimes if two caregivers work closely with each other they tend to support the others' decisions, even if they do have some reservations. By seeing someone unfamiliar with your original caregiver you may get a more impartial assessment of your condition.

Asking About Mental Health Care

When first interviewing a mental health professional such as a psychiatric social worker, psychiatrist, or psychologist, you should keep in mind that there is considerable debate among caregivers as to which is the most effective treatment for many emotional difficulties. Some prefer to use medication while others use counseling. One basic principle in your search for high quality care should be to find a place where both medication and counseling are available to you if you need them. Before you make an office visit, your potential caregiver should be willing to talk about such medical and psychological treatment options with you.

Because each of these treatments requires special expertise, it may be in your best interest to be treated where there are specialized professionals. When you meet with a mental health practitioner for the first time, you may want to ask about the other caregivers with whom that professional regularly consults. Does the caregiver have access to a psychiatrist, for example, who might be able to rule out the possibility that a medical disorder is the root of your problem? Is it possible for the caregiver to talk with a psychologist who could recommend ways to help you increase your self-control or manage your anger? Is a social worker available to assist in your search for better housing or find free legal advice? Asking these questions will help you get a better idea if your caregiver has help from others with different types of training and expertise. Even if you are working with someone who works alone the person should still know about other professionals in the community to turn to for help.

Rather than describe in any detail the hundreds of therapies that are used in the field of mental health, I will mention just a few of the most common treatments. First, medications are being prescribed more often these days for many problems. These include such common concerns as depression, anxiety, and fears. In addition, drugs are used for less frequently occurring difficulties such as "schizophrenia," where people have symptoms such as hallucinations, bizarre behavior, and inappropriate speech or unusual beliefs. Other problems often treated with medication include "bipolar disorder," which may include quick changes from excited and loud behavior to periods of severe depression. Each of these problems, as well as many others, are frequently treated effectively with medication. Although psychiatrists often are the ones who give such medications, other general physicians who have not specialized in mental health care also commonly prescribe some of these drugs.

If medication is recommended, be sure to ask questions about its side effects, just as you would for pills prescribed for any other ailment. Some drugs, for example, that are used to control schizophrenia produce an often permanent problem called "tardive dyskinesia." People having this disorder may eventually show permanent uncontrollable writhing of the limbs along with involuntary facial movements that may include sucking, sticking out the tongue, or grimacing. Often these symptoms can be prevented or kept to a minimum by the physician who carefully monitors the appearance of symptoms and keeps medication dosages low. Some medications used to treat psychological problems are dangerous to take when you eat certain foods or are given other drugs at the same time. Others cause symptoms such as dry mouth, feelings of "unreality," difficulty concentrating, or feelings of losing control. With proper medical care however, many of these symptoms can usually be controlled. And, in spite of such side effects in some people, the drugs are often very helpful in the treatment of emotional difficulties.

"Talk therapies" usually involve regular meetings, usually 50 minutes long, with a mental health professional. Typically these are scheduled once each week for people who are not confined to a hospital. People often meet more frequently with their caregiver if they are hospitalized or in greater distress. These days mental health professionals usually use a variety of techniques to help people during these sessions. One method is referred to as "behavior therapy." With this therapy people are encouraged to change their behavior by learning new skills and/or by earning rewards. For example, a couple who wants to improve their marriage could be helped to alter specific behaviors. Here, they may learn to express affection more often or in different ways, they may be taught to resolve arguments and communicate with each other more effectively, or they may learn to talk calmly with each other about who should carry out certain household duties. Changes in each of these areas by one person often are rewarded by a favor of some type from the spouse. By using other therapies professionals may encourage people to express their emotions and, sometimes, to look for the origins of these emotions in things that happened many years earlier. Some other techniques involve helping people to find ways to change current beliefs that cause emotional difficulties. Sometimes these beliefs are termed "irrational" and people are helped to examine more critically the logic that underlies them.

In certain situations, each of these and many other kinds of counseling are effective. For the past thirty years or so there has been a tremendous amount of scientific research on the effectiveness of different forms of therapy. The researchers are now to the point where they usually have a reasonable idea about how effective a given therapy is for psychological problems. When you first talk with the mental health professional then, you can ask about how effective the research has shown this particular drug or counseling technique to be with your problem. If you ask specific questions (for example about the percentage of people who recover) you are likely to get much more of a feel for both the probability of recovery and for your therapist's knowledge of this scientific literature. Also, ask yourself if you like the professional you might be working with. In the field of mental health it's usually vital that you are comfortable with your caregiver and that you feel free to discuss problems that may be personal.

Before you work with a mental health professional, be sure to have them describe in some detail how they usually treat people with your problem. Then ask yourself if that plan makes sense and is a form of therapy that you would probably be comfortable with.

What's right for one person might go against the grain of another. And, if you don't like the methods used by your mental health professional, they most likely won't help you.

You should also be aware that counseling makes some psychological symptoms worse. As with medication, it can have harmful side effects. In one excellent review of many studies (Bergin & Lambert, 1978) the authors concluded that a "deterioration effect" is a significant problem for individual psychotherapy. They noted that people receiving therapies that expose them to frightening objects or situations, (as often happens to people treated for phobias), have sometimes become depressed (Marks, 1971). Group counseling may also produce casualties. Perhaps it is most common for this to occur when a group leader is very direct and aggressive with group members without being sensitive to the ability of group members to tolerate this confrontation. Bergin and Lambert referred to one particular study (Yalom & Leiberman, 1971) that quoted a confrontational leader who remarked:

> *...it was a stubborn group, full of people too infantile to take responsibility for themselves and to form an adult contract...I saw that most of the group didn't want to do anything so what I did was to just go ahead and have a good time for myself.*

This kind of recklessness can be terribly destructive to people who are genuinely seeking help. This leader's attitude is especially unfortunate because group therapy is often quite helpful if it is carried out by a skilled therapist who is looking out for the best interests of group members.

Other researchers have studied deterioration in encounter groups where people are put "on the spot" and challenged by other group members. In one study, Lieberman, Yalom, and Miles (1973) found that almost ten percent of the people that fully participated in these groups suffered "significant psychological injury." Many of these people actually needed psychotherapy to repair the damage they suffered in the groups. A number of caregivers have remarked that the Food and Drug Administration would never allow any medication to be sold that injured ten percent of the people who used it. If these confrontational psychotherapies were subject to this same standard, they would be illegal.

If you think you are suffering because of psychotherapy, talk about your concerns with your therapist. You may also want to discuss the matter with the professional organization to which your therapist belongs. They may be able to offer an impartial opinion and, if necessary, send you to another caregiver.

As with all other health problems, be sure to "shop around" and talk to a number of caregivers before you make your final decision. The mental health professionals you interview will most likely have different types of training and professional degrees. This will help you learn more about the many treatments that are available from a wide range of caregivers in your community.

Choosing a Hospital

If your health insurance plan allows you to choose your own hospital, your selection may play a large role in determining whether or not you receive competent care. This is because the quality of service can vary from one facility to the next. Some hospitals don't have the sophisticated equipment necessary to diagnose or treat certain illnesses. Others have poorly trained staff and few specialists. And some have administrators who may be more interested in making profits than in providing quality care.

A recent study (Hartz, et al., 1989) of over three thousand U.S. hospitals suggests that problems like these may result in increased death rates in many facilities. The authors of this study found that the training of the physicians and nurses was closely related to hospital deaths. Those hospitals that did best were those that had a higher percentage of specialists. The more successful hospitals also had more R.N.'s. These are not surprising results because practitioners with longer, more extensive training are likely to provide better care.

Another finding was that hospitals that had many doctors of osteopathy (D.O.) tended to have higher mortality rates. This statistic will certainly cause considerable debate. Here, some groups will likely claim that this study shows the care provided by M.D.'s is superior to that given by osteopaths.

Hospitals also had lower death rates if they were financially stable. Presumably, this allowed the hospital to spend more money on treatment for each consumer. For example, the financially healthy hospital might be able to provide more customers with private nurses who could pay closer attention to their needs. Hospitals that were larger and had more technologically sophisticated equipment also fared better. The benefits of size and up-to-date machinery seemed to give them the advantage over smaller hospitals who generally had fewer resources.

Finally, the study looked at several different kinds of hospitals. The first of these, called "private for-profit" hospitals, are generally owned by private corporations. They are run with the primary goal of making a profit, just like other businesses. The second type of hospital, public hospitals, are owned and supported by taxpayers. Commonly these are financed by city or county funds as are all government institutions. Public hospitals are the hospitals that people who have little money are likely to visit. This is because these facilities may not require payment if a person has financial problems or no health insurance. The study found that both of these types of hospitals (private for-profit and public) had higher death rates than a third kind of hospital, called "private not-for-profit." Private not-for-profit hospitals are privately owned and not supported by the government. Their goals differ from those of for-profit hospitals in that they are not attempting to make money for investors, only to provide care to customers.

The fact that for-profit hospitals had higher death rates than not-for-profit hospitals has been interpreted by many to mean that facilities that try to make money may be less concerned with maintaining a high quality of care. Instead, they might be paying more attention to the well-being of their stockholders who demand dividends on their investments.

The news that public hospitals seem to have less success keeping their customers alive is probably especially distressing to minority groups and the poor. They tend to use these institutions more often because they may be unable to afford private facilities. The higher death rates in these hospitals are sometimes blamed on both the government's lack of commitment to high quality care and to dwindling funds.

The hospitals that had the lowest death rates were private "teaching hospitals." These facilities are partly designed as schools for those who are learning to provide health care services. They are frequently associated with a private university. The university students visit hospitalized people and provide treatment under the supervision of fully qualified practitioners. Quite often these are the facilities where you are likely to be visited by legions of young health care professionals who all want to learn about your illness.

If you do choose to go to a teaching hospital, keep in mind that you may be working with some "doc-lings" who have just received their medical degrees. The greenest of these, referred to as "interns," often begin working in teaching hospitals during the month of June. There is considerable debate as to whether or not hospital customers get poorer care during this month. Some evidence shows that people who are treated by newer interns tend to stay in the hospital a bit longer than people whose interns are more experienced. People treated by more seasoned interns though don't seem to live longer or do better after leaving the hospital than do people whose caregivers have less experience (Rich, Gifford, Luxenberg, & Dowd, 1990).

Other writers (Schuman, 1990) argue that new M.D.'s just don't have the experience needed to skillfully perform certain procedures. For example, one study (Eisenhauer, Derveloy, & Hastings, 1982) looked at how often people suffered from complications as a result of having a catheter placed in one of their major blood vessels. Those researchers found that complications happened almost three times as often if the catheters were inserted by less experienced physicians. Other research has shown that some inexperienced surgeons have had poorer results when doing certain difficult types of ear surgery (Vernick, 1986). These physician's customers were especially likely to suffer from complications such as torn eardrums or facial weakness.

Perhaps the best advice to those in any hospital is to be especially cautious when being treated by less experienced caregivers. Not only would this include physicians, but also students in many other fields such as physical therapy, psychology, and speech pathology. For those treated in teaching hospitals, caution may be even more important during July and the next few months. It is at this time that many new M.D.'s may be on the scene who are just beginning to develop their skills.

When choosing a hospital, it's also important to know how many people with your illness have already been treated in that hospital. A number of studies (Eastaugh, 1986) have suggested that people are much more likely to survive surgery if they are staying in a hospital that has treated many people in the past with similar difficulties. In fact, one study (Maerki, Luft, & Hunt, 1986) found that 61% of the deaths that resulted from hysterectomy in some hospitals could have been avoided if people had gone to hospitals where physicians had been more experienced in doing that surgery. Another interesting finding (Flood, Scott & Ewy, 1984) was that hospitals with more experience kept more of their customers alive even if the surgery was relatively simple. In other words, the experienced hospitals were more successful, even when doing operations that were not very difficult. The hospital you select should be willing to provide you with precise statistics on their success treating people with your particular problem. If they seem reluctant or refuse, you may want to go somewhere else.

To help consumers in their search for high quality care, the U.S. government has published statistics on mortality rates from thousands of hospitals. This report identifies those facilities that have the highest mortality rates. One problem with this report though is that it doesn't take into account the fact that some hospitals may simply have had sicker customers to work with. The more serious illnesses, not poor care, may have resulted in that hospital having a higher than average death rate. Nevertheless, these statistics are probably useful to the consumer who wants to look for potential problems with a particular facility. If a hospital has too many customers die, the consumer may at least want to consider going to another facility.

If you would like copies of this government report, entitled "Medicare Hospital Mortality Information," write to the Government Printing Office, Washington, D. C., 20402. The report will cost around $70. Otherwise, you might call your state health department or local hospital association and get the same information at no charge. Each of these organizations has been sent a copy of this report and should be able to give you the information you need over the telephone.

Keep in mind that the mortality rate will probably not be your only consideration when choosing a hospital. You could be more concerned about other things such as a particular specialty service it may offer. It's likely that death rates do reflect something about the general level of care available in the different types of facilities though. And consequently, it may be worthwhile for you to keep this information in mind when you make your selection, no matter what your priorities are.

Many people prefer going to a hospital that is near friends and relatives. If this true with you, remember that there are lots of things to consider when selecting a hospital other than just how convenient it is for people to visit you there. Although it may be calming for you to have these people nearby, remember that your first priority is to receive quality health care. And, the closest hospital is not necessarily the one that is best equipped to deliver this service. Therefore you may have to sacrifice frequent visits by loved ones in order to have better treatment at a hospital that is farther away from your home.

Also, some people go to the hospital recommended by their caregivers without first verifying that it is the facility in the area best equipped to treat their illnesses. This is very dangerous because many caregivers recommend only one or two hospitals simply to make it possible for them to earn more money. It's more profitable for them to spend their time treating people in one place than to waste time driving from one hospital to the next. So again, be sure to question almost all recommendations made by caregivers, even their choice of hospitals.

Fortunately, most hospitals are under the watchful eye of the Joint Commission on Accreditation of Healthcare Organizations (JCAHO) a private organization that monitors the quality of care in hospitals with twenty-five or more beds. A hospital is eligible to be inspected by JCAHO every three years. Many insurance companies require that hospitals pass this inspection before they pay the hospital for care provided to their subscribers. JCAHO inspects the basic organization of health care in the hospital as well as record keeping. In so doing, it helps insure that its customers receive high quality treatment. If a hospital meets the standards of JCAHO, it receives a certificate of accreditation. If a hospital has not been awarded this certificate, you may want to consider going elsewhere for your care. You can find out if a particular hospital has been approved by JCAHO by looking for their accreditation certificate posted near the entrances or by calling the hospital's general information line. Another alternative is to call JCAHO directly at (708) 916-5600.

In many areas of the country insurance plans have had a major impact on the quality of the hospital care. To reduce costs, many of these plans have negotiated with hospitals to provide discounts for their own subscribers. In this arrangement, all people with that type of insurance are sent to one hospital. This guarantees the hospital a steady supply of customers. In return, the hospital agrees to give the insurance plan a discount in the price they pay for their customers' hospital care. In other words, the insurer is allowed to pay less money to the hospital for your care because, in exchange, it sends the hospital business.

Because the hospital collects less insurance money for each customer it may be forced to cut expenses. Hospitals, like other businesses, have to make at least as much money as they spend in order to stay afloat. Hospitals may cut costs in a variety of ways. Perhaps one of the most common is to eliminate the jobs of those hospital employees who make less profit for the hospital. This might include chaplains, groundskeepers, security personnel, and so forth. Such people generally do not directly charge hospital customers for their services and, at the same time, they cost the hospital money. When people employed in these jobs are laid off, however, quality of customer care often suffers because the services are no longer available. When you decide to bring your business to a certain hospital, you may want to see if it will be able to offer you access to the services of all the different professionals that should be involved in your care. It is likely that these will be the institutions that are most stable financially and will therefore be able to spend more on your care. Those that are having financial problems on the other hand are more likely to cut corners and offer poorer quality treatment.

The following list, based partly on the study by Hartz et al., is provided to help you remember some of the important questions to ask when selecting a hospital.

Hospital Quality Checklist

1. Does it provide all of the specialists I may need? (It may be easiest to ask your primary caregiver this question, assuming that he or she is familiar with the hospital.)
2. Are the staff highly trained compared to other hospitals in the area? Again, your primary caregiver might be of help here. You might also call the hospital to ask about the qualifications of different professionals. For example, you may ask about how many of the physicians are "board certified" or what degrees and training the nurses have that are likely to provide your care.
3. Is it financially stable? You might have some idea of this if it has laid off employees recently, has closed parts of its facility, or seems to be cutting back service in other areas. If you are a bit daring, you might even call someone in the hospital administration to see if the hospital is making money or is in debt.
4. Is it public or private? Remember, private hospitals sometimes have lower death rates.
5. Is it a teaching hospital? They may have lower death rates if they are also private.
6. Is this hospital a not-for-profit organization? They are sometimes associated with lower death rates than hospitals that are out to earn money for investors.
7. Are there a large number of osteopaths practicing in this hospital? Again, the controversial finding that osteopaths seem to be associated with somewhat higher death rates may influence some people's choice of hospital.
8. Is this hospital approved by the Joint Commission on

Accreditation of Healthcare Organizations? Look for a certificate in the entrance of the hospital, call the hospital administration, or contact JCAHO for this information.

9. Is this hospital large enough and does it have the sophisticated equipment that I may need? Again, your health care practitioner will be able to answer this question best.
10. Has this hospital treated a large number of people with my illness? Remember, practice makes perfect.

CHAPTER 3

Insurance

"Never let those ruby slippers off your feet for a moment, or you will be at the mercy of the Wicked Witch of the West."

—Glinda, the Good Witch
(The Wizard Of OZ, *1939*)

Fee-For-Service Insurance

With health care costs today as high as they are, few people can afford to risk not being covered by a good health insurance policy. Bills totaling tens of thousands of dollars can pile up easily after just a few weeks in the hospital. Those who don't have good insurance may find themselves deep in debt or forced to hold bake sales to pay for their appendectomies. Just as bad, some of those same people may find themselves at institutions that offer poorer quality care because they cannot pay for treatment at better facilities. Others go without treatment. Two-thirds of people with hypertension, for example, don't receive effective treatment, largely because the medications are too expensive ("Crisis in Health," 1990).

Traditional "fee-for-service" health insurance plans ask you to pay a set fee in exchange for guaranteed coverage of health care expenses. Caregivers are reimbursed each time they provide you with treatment. Under these plans, you are sometimes free to go to any qualified caregivers and are not limited to those who practice in a certain clinic or geographic location. This is one advantage that these plans often have over health maintenance organizations (HMO's). With HMO's you may face much more severe restrictions about where you can receive your health care.

These fee-for-service policies usually charge you a "deductible" fee for your care. For example, you may be responsible for the first $500 of your health care bills each year. After paying that deductible out of your pocket, the health plan will cover a percentage of the rest of your "eligible" expenses. The example below illustrates what might happen with a typical fee-for-service insurance plan.

Here, if a caregiver charges you $1000 for ten treatments, the insurance plan might state that only $700 will be considered to be "eligible" expenses. They determine eligible expenses by calculating what the customary fees are of other caregivers in your community. Then you might be responsible for paying a deductible. This could easily amount to the first $500 of that $700 of eligible expenses. The insurance company would then pay a percentage, let's say 80%, of the remaining $200. The $40 that is left is considered to be your co-payment of 20%. This means that the insurance company eventually pays only $160 of the original $1000 charge. Your total payment amounts to $840. Deductibles, co-payments, and low "eligible" expenses then are probably the major disadvantages of fee-for-service plans. Although you may have greater freedom to choose your provider with fee-for-service insurance, it may cost you more money.

$1000 = (YOUR ORIGINAL BILL)
-$300 = The insurance company decides the caregiver overcharged you by $300. You are responsible for paying this excess.

THIS LEAVES:
$700 = "eligible" expenses.
-$500 = Because you have a $500 deductible you pay the first $500 of this amount.

THIS LEAVES:
$200 of which the insurance company will pay 80%...
$160 = (80% of $200)
$40 = (Your 20% co-payment)

WHAT THE INSURANCE COMPANY PAYS = $160.00
WHAT YOU PAY = $840.00

The greater freedom of choice offered by fee-for-service policies, however, may be changing. Some of these plans now encourage consumers to see only caregivers who are enrolled as "participating providers." These professionals have agreed to accept, as payment in full, the amount of money that the insurance plan decides is a "reasonable and customary" charge. They are not allowed to bill consumers for charges that the insurance plan will not cover. Consumers are usually required to pay lower deductibles if they are cared for by these practitioners. The insurance company also saves because they pay participating providers less than they pay those who are not enrolled. The advantage to the caregivers participating in the plan is that they are more likely to see new people who want to take advantage of the lower deductibles. One unfortunate consequence of this is that the insurance plan is making it more expensive for you to see non participating providers, thus limiting your freedom of choice. Obviously such advantages and disadvantages of HMO's and traditional fee-for-service insurance need to be considered when selecting an insurance plan.

Through your job you may be able to find the best traditional insurance plan. These plans often offer better coverage and require you to pay lower deductibles. In addition, many employers will pay for a portion of your health insurance, a benefit that may save you money. If you are a member of a trade union or a professional group you might also be able to find a good value for your health care dollar by purchasing a plan through one of those organizations.

Before you buy health insurance, be sure to anticipate your own health care needs. Do you expect that you will need care in a nursing home for a long time? What mental health care are you likely to use? You can even make a list of the treatment you may need in the future. Use this list when asking the representative from the insurance company about the fee-for-service policy you are considering purchasing. Below are some of the questions you might ask:

1. How much does the policy cost?
2. What deductible (if any) would I be required to pay for:
   a. Medication?
   b. Visits to a physician?
   c. Mental health care?
   d. Dental work?

e. Hospital room charges?
f. Eye care and eye glasses
3. After the deductible is paid, what percentage of the expenses will the insurance company pay?
4. Does the policy use "select" and "ultimate" rates to determine my premiums? Some companies initially charge low (select) rates to new customers who are in good health. A few years later the company hikes up their rates to the highest (ultimate) level.
5. Is this a "dread-disease" or "hospital-indemnity" policy? (Dread-disease policies only pay when you contract a specific disease such as cancer or heart disease. Hospital-indemnity policies pay only a fixed amount when you are hospitalized. Each is a bad buy for most consumers.)
6. Can the insurance company cancel the policy or am I guaranteed to be able to renew it for the rest of my life?
7. Is nursing home care covered? For how long?
8. Is treatment for drug or alcohol dependence covered?
9. How much paperwork will I have to do to file a claim?
10. Will I pay a lower deductible if I am treated by a participating provider?
11. Are physical exams covered even if I don't have a problem?
12. Will treatment for a problem I had before enrolling in this insurance plan be covered?
13. Will I still be able to work with the caregivers who have treated me in the past?
14. What are the maximum benefits paid by this policy for each type of health care I might need?
15. Can I continue my group insurance policy or convert it to an individual plan if my job ends? If so, will it cost more and will the coverage change? (This question might apply if you are thinking of enrolling in a group insurance plan through your job or another organization)

Health Maintenance Organizations

In the past few years there have been many different types of health insurance plans available for consumers. These have included plans offered through "preferred provider organizations" (PPO's,) "health maintenance organizations" (HMO's,) as well as other specialized health care packages tailored for specific company's employees. All of these plans have their own merits and their own problems. Because there are so many new types of insurance, it is impossible to describe each in this book. Perhaps the most common kinds of plans though, and the ones that seem to have many of the advantages and disadvantages so typical of the others, are offered by HMO's.

HMO's are a relatively recent development that largely came about in an effort to reduce the costs of health care in the United States. This cost reduction has been necessary because of the tremendous increase in the price of health care. Health care expenses are expected to increase by more than 10 percent a year through the 1990s. Prices are rising so quickly that many people are predicting that in the near future decent health insurance will no longer be routinely provided by employers because it will cost too much. Employers go to great lengths to lower their costs and help their employees stay healthy. Many large corporations, for example, spend millions of dollars on health club memberships. They have found that the most physically fit employees often spend less on medical care and miss fewer work days (Bly, Jones, & Richardson, 1986; Blair, Piserchia, Wilbur, & Crowder, 1986). One company, an ice cream manufacturer, has a particularly innovative program. Not only do their employees receive complimentary memberships in health clubs, but they also are given massage for stress relief and free ice cream.

Some employers have already resorted to less appealing tactics to reduce their health care costs. For example, some screen new employees and their family members and charge them higher premiums if they have significant preexisting health problems. Some even refuse to hire employees who smoke. This is because employees who smoke may eventually cost the employer money as they often have more health problems and miss more work than nonsmokers.

Employers have also turned to HMO's for alternatives to the

expensive insurance they have purchased for their employees in the past. One innovative method HMO's have used to cut costs has been to place more emphasis on prevention of illness. One such program was developed by Group Health, Inc., a Minneapolis HMO that designed a Preterm Birth Program ("Program lowers, 1986") to reduce the risk of premature delivery. Babies born prematurely can cost hundreds of thousands of dollars to keep alive. Later in life they may have many other costly problems such as mental retardation, cerebral palsy, and blindness. Understandably, it is in the HMO's best interest to reduce their own costs by insuring that their enrollees have the best chance possible of having normal full-term pregnancies.

Group Health's program involves first surveying expectant mothers to identify those at high risk to deliver prematurely. Their survey questions women about their medical histories and current life-styles. The survey also asks about drug and alcohol use, work habits, and social stress because problems in each of these areas may make it more likely that a woman will deliver early. Women identified as high risk are then given the chance to take classes designed to lower their chances of premature birth.

In these classes women are taught to recognize the signs of preterm labor. This includes learning what labor feels like as well as remembering to check for contractions. They are encouraged to call their practitioner at the first sign of trouble. Also, women are taught how to deal with stress and to use the support systems available in their community. The results of this program have been quite encouraging. The number of premature births in class graduates is approximately half the national average. Even the babies that are born early to mothers in this program seem to have higher birth weights. These results mean both healthier babies for HMO customers and tremendous financial savings for the HMO.

In order to understand some of the other strategies HMO's use to lower the cost of health care, it is necessary to know how HMO's operate financially. If you are a member of an HMO you pay a set fee and, in return, your health care costs are covered. Your monthly fee does not increase, even if you need expensive care. This means that when you are treated, the HMO does not get paid extra for providing that treatment. Instead, your care costs the HMO money. It is in the financial interest of the HMO, then, for you to need as little care as possible. This way the HMO collects the same amount of money while it pays for less treatment.

This is similar to health clubs turning a profit. With both HMO's and health clubs it is most lucrative for the company to receive monthly payments from people who seldom take advantage of the services offered. With the health club, you may be offered unlimited use of the physical fitness equipment. After you have joined, however, you are probably not encouraged to use the pool or the other facilities. This is because if everyone who belonged to your health club used it regularly, it would be too crowded and soon forced out of business. Similarly, the HMO doesn't encourage you to make extra office visits that would cost them money and reduce their profits. Of course, this is also similar to how traditional fee-for-service insurance plans operate. Each bets that the people they insure will not need expensive care.

The professionals who work in an HMO are often salaried employees whose paychecks do not increase if they treat people more frequently. There is no financial incentive for those caregivers to encourage consumers to make unnecessary office visits. This saves HMO's (and ultimately consumers!) money. Other professionals employed by HMO's are paid partly on a profit-sharing basis. This means that when the HMO makes more money it is shared with the caregivers. This may create a strong incentive for your health care provider to treat you fewer times in order to increase his or her own paycheck. In other words, the less you are treated the more money providers make.

It is also common for HMO's to reward their caregivers with bonuses at the end of the year for spending less of the HMO's money. If fact, practitioners who cost the HMO more might actually risk their own job security. The result is that many caregivers working in HMO's cut costs by ordering fewer medical tests, seeing people for fewer visits, and discouraging customers from working with other specialists.

A 1986 U.S. federal law made it illegal to these incentive systems to pressure caregivers working for hospitals to spend less money on customer care (Millenson, 1990). Congress has also considered stopping HMO's from paying practitioners more if they treat customers for less money. At the time of this writing though, it is uncertain as to whether or not such a ban will actually occur. Even if this happens though, HMO's will probably still be able to force caregivers to cut costs. Instead of rewarding them for spending less, they may be fired if they spend too much (Pauly, in Millenson, 1990).

It is not a bad idea to encourage professionals to think before they recommend expensive health care. After all, many of the treatments prescribed today are unnecessary or dangerous as well as costly (Leape, 1989). For example, one recent study (Hillman, et al., 1990) showed that physicians take more than four times as many X-rays if they own the X-ray machines and make a profit on them. Clearly, this may result in many people being needlessly exposed to radiation and to increased health care costs. Other problems occur, though, when people are discouraged from finding care they need. Louis Zako M.D. (Zako, 1989) for example, has said that a few physicians will try to save HMO's money by avoiding necessary surgery. Dr. Zako also pointed out that some HMO physicians perform exams quickly in order to increase their own productivity and their own paychecks.[2] Finally, he complains consumers wait up to two months for referrals to specialists. Each of these practices increases HMO profits by discouraging consumers from using health care services that should, in fact, be readily available.[3]

Though these cost-saving tactics are healthy for the HMO,

2 — Of course, this also happens with professionals paid by fee-for-service insurance plans. The more people they see, the more bills they can send out.

3 — This is similar to the problems faced by some consumers in Great Britain. There, health care is often rationed. This sometimes means that expensive treatment, even if medically necessary, is not given to the people who need it. For example, some older people are denied kidney dialysis. As a result of this they die. Caregivers have been forced to only treat younger people because it would cost too much to treat everyone who needed care. It's interesting to see how caregivers in Great Britain sometimes justify withholding such treatment from older people. This is often done by emphasizing the negative consequences of treatment or by being generally pessimistic about the chances of recovery. One caregiver even claimed that "everyone over the age of 55 is a bit crumbly" anyway (Aaron & Schwartz, 1990).

let's look at their possible effects on the consumer. Consider routine blood screening. Such testing, although expensive, may be necessary to diagnose many rare medical problems. Instead of checking for all of those unlikely problems, the physician might ask that the blood be screened only for the few diseases that you are most likely to have. This will cost the HMO less money because more tests have not been done. How many times might omitting such "extra" tests prevent the discovery of real problems?

This is a difficult question. Whether or not omitting some routine tests really affects the quality of care can be difficult to determine. It may be that doing without many less important (and sometimes dangerous) tests will prevent people from being exposed to unnecessary risk. HMO's that provide high quality care usually see to it that the most important and less risky tests are given routinely. This is to assure that consumers are checked for the most common illnesses while keeping the danger to a minimum.

One study of some other effects of HMO cost-saving tactics (Hillman, Pauly, & Kerstein, 1989) showed that physicians in HMO's were less likely to hospitalize people if there was no financial reward to them for doing so. These were HMO physicians who were either on fixed salaries or were paid a set amount for each person, no matter what care was provided. Also, physicians who practiced in HMO's that were in business to make a profit were apparently more reluctant to spend the HMO's money by keeping people in the hospital. The results of this study also suggested that physicians who were penalized for costing the HMO more seemed to encourage their customers to make fewer office visits. Although it was not proved by this study, these findings suggest that a few HMO caregivers may be trying to cut corners. If the incentives are right, their customers visit their offices less frequently and spend fewer days in the hospital.

Consider another example of how some HMO's try to keep their costs low. To do this, let's look at mental health care. Members of an HMO needing counseling will often meet for an hour each week with a professional such as a psychiatric social worker, a psychologist, or a psychiatrist. These caregivers usually spend 20 to 30 hours every week doing individual, marital, and family counseling with different HMO subscribers. Often it is necessary for these professionals to meet with a subscriber for many weeks, even years, to insure proper treatment. Many people have long histories of depression, marital problems, and drug or alcohol abuse that may require many visits to a counselor. Unfortunately such long term treatment can be very costly to an HMO. Instead, it saves the HMO money if the client is treated with fewer counseling sessions.

To encourage mental health professionals to treat people in less time, HMO's may tell caregivers to work regularly with many new people. For example, a psychiatric social worker might be told to see six new clients weekly. This is in addition to the social worker's eighteen hours of counseling with his or her previous clients. On the average, this would result in this professional treating clients only four hours each before bringing therapy to an end. This arrangement discourages working with one person for a long time even though that person may need many years of treatment. Some people believe that such a system emphasizes quicker turnover at the expense of quality care.

Another way HMO's sometimes have to spend extra money is when one of their own practitioners cannot provide your treatment. This might happen when you need a specialized type of surgery that only a few surgeons are trained to perform. If the HMO does not employ a surgeon with those skills they are still obligated to pay for your treatment. This means that they have to send you to a surgeon who is not a member of their HMO. Remember, if one of their own surgeons treated you it would have been less expensive for the HMO. This is because that surgeon already may have been on the HMO's fixed salary. The non HMO surgeon on the other hand, may charge the HMO thousands of dollars more to perform the operation.

If you need such a surgeon, your HMO has two options. First, it can agree to refer you to the physician who is not a member of your HMO but who is well qualified to perform your surgery. This will insure that you receive the best care. Fortunately this is the decision that most HMO's make. Less frequently, HMO's decide to save money by refusing to send you to non HMO surgeons. Instead, they insist that one of their own physicians will perform your surgery. This way the HMO avoids paying an "outside" provider. Unfortunately, the HMO physician might have had very little experience doing the kind of operation that you need.

The HMO also may be interested in helping their own physician gain experience by doing your surgery. By working on you, this surgeon might learn to operate more skillfully on future HMO subscribers. If this happens, the HMO physician should at least have done enough of the surgeries to technically be qualified to do your operation. Even with this experience, though, this physician probably will not be very skilled. Here, this practitioner could have performed five or ten of the surgeries while the non HMO surgeon down the hall may have done hundreds. Although the HMO surgeon could do an adequate job, the other physician might have had much better results because of the benefit of having had more practice. Unfortunately, if a problem happens because of your surgeon's lack of experience, you may not find out until it's too late to correct it.

Therefore, the cost of sending you to a non HMO practitioner may present a great ethical problem for your HMO. On the one hand, it is obligated to send you to an outside professional if there is nobody working within the HMO who is qualified to treat your problem. On the other hand, if you are referred elsewhere, the HMO loses money.

Let's contrast the incentives of HMO health professionals with those of providers paid by traditional health insurance plans. Remember that with fee-for-service insurance, professionals are paid more each time they treat you. This sometimes creates an incentive for them to provide unnecessary and sometimes even dangerous treatment. So, while the person covered by an HMO may need to be aware of a tendency for caregivers to provide too little treatment, people with fee-for-service plans may need to be more watchful of practitioners who provide excessive treatment.

With traditional fee-for-service insurance plans, however, it can be easier for you to get more treatment when you need it.

Again, this is because when you are treated more frequently your health provider makes more money. It is also often easier for you to be treated by a wider variety of health professionals. This is because the traditional health insurance plans will usually pay for professional services even though the professional is not a member of an HMO or a similar organization. In other words, you can shop all over town for the help you need instead of being restricted to the HMO professionals. Remember, though, that one drawback of fee-for-service insurance plans is that they are often more expensive. Increased costs may be reflected in higher monthly insurance premiums, higher co-payments that require you to pay a fee each time you see a practitioner, limited "eligible" expenses, or higher deductibles. They also may encourage caregivers to perform unnecessary or even dangerous treatment.

What do you do if you are dissatisfied with the quality of care your HMO professional offers? You may have worked with both of the audiologists employed by your HMO and were dissatisfied with the help they gave you for your hearing difficulties. With traditional insurance you could usually shop around until you found an audiologist who met your standards. But with an HMO that employs only a few audiologists, you have few choices. The HMO will probably refuse to pay for services with an outside audiologist, claiming their own employees can meet your needs.

One option is to complain to the HMO about the quality of care you received. Be specific about why you are dissatisfied. You might also argue that an outside audiologist is uniquely qualified to help you with your particular difficulty. This would be the case if the audiologists in your HMO didn't have the training to diagnose an uncommon hearing problem from which you suffer. In a rare instance you may threaten a lawsuit if you believe that you will be harmed by not getting specialized care from a non HMO professional. More often than not though these moves only work if you can make a very strong argument that another caregiver will give you better service.

The important thing to remember is do not take for granted you have the best health care provider just because he or she is highly recommended by an HMO. Investigate that person's credentials and experience and make your own decision.

I recall one person's experience bargaining with an HMO. Orlando had been diagnosed as having a small tumor on the nerve that came from his ear. This tumor could only be removed safely by someone who had much skill and experience. A botched job could cause many lifelong problems, including paralyzed muscles in his face and chronic headaches. None of the surgeons in his HMO had removed this kind of tumor before. Because of this, the HMO was forced to refer Orlando to a non HMO surgeon.

The surgeon the HMO recommended happened to practice in a nearby hospital. They said this physician was "well qualified" but was also trying to gain experience doing this surgery. During Orlando's first appointment, this physician said he had performed 35 of these operations. He said that the procedure often took him, working with a team of other surgeons, more than ten hours. This physician also said that he would schedule the operation as soon as he could "dig up" a team of surgeons to assist.

After this meeting, Orlando was uncomfortable with the surgeon the HMO recommended. Not only did he make putting together a surgical team sound like starting a game of pick-up basketball, but he didn't have quite enough experience. With some research in the library, Orlando found the clinic where this surgery had originally been developed. The physicians there had performed more than three thousand of these operations and rarely needed to spend more than three hours on each. They also used the same surgeons for each customer so they would always have only the most experienced people performing the operation.

At first, the HMO said it would not to pay for the surgery if it was done by the more experienced group of physicians. The HMO representative said that the other surgeons, although admittedly more skilled, practiced in a state that had a reputation for over-charging for medical care. After a week or so, however, the HMO said it would be flexible and "consented" to pay $7000, even if Orlando decided to have the procedure done elsewhere. The HMO also claimed that the $7000 should cover most of the expenses and would make it possible for him to go wherever he wanted for his treatment.

With some checking, Orlando learned that the charges would probably exceed $18,000 anywhere in the United States, including at the hospital the HMO originally suggested. A written estimate from the out-of-state clinic, in fact, was almost identical to that from the in-state facility. When confronted with this, the HMO agreed to pay 80% of the bill at the hospital of his choice.

There were a number of lessons Orlando learned from this experience. First, he found out that he could bargain with his HMO. Their "decision" to refuse to pay for his surgery out of state was not a final decision after all, but just their first position. When faced with the true cost of the procedure the HMO had no choice but to offer to pay for the surgery elsewhere. This experience also drove home the point that the HMO seemed to be as concerned with their own financial profits as they were with his quality of care. In the end, Orlando saw that he was able to receive high quality health care through the HMO, but not without effort. It just took some assertiveness on his part along with a basic understanding of the HMO's financial concerns.

The problems with HMO's do not mean that you need to turn to fee-for-service insurance to receive high quality health care. Excellent care is usually provided by HMO's and by other new types of insurance plans. However, problems sometimes result when consumers don't know enough about the strategies insurers use to control costs, occasionally at the expense of quality treatment. This puts even more of a burden on people to be informed consumers who keep track of their own care.

Before you join an HMO, ask questions about the health care it provides and the costs of belonging to the plan. Below are a number of questions that may be helpful for you to consider.

1. What kinds of incentives are there, if any, for the caregivers in this HMO to keep treatment costs low?
2. How many health care providers (such as physicians, dentists, or other specialists) belong to your HMO? (This will tell you how many caregivers are available to choose from if you join.)
3. What permission, if any, do I need to get a second opinion or to see a specialist?

4. Will I see the same caregiver every visit or will I have to see the professional that happens to be assigned to me that day? (In some HMO's, consumers may see a different caregiver every visit, depending on who happens to be available the day of their appointment.)
5. Could I have a list of the caregivers that work in your HMO along with information about the schools from which they received their professional degrees?
6. What hospitals will the HMO allow me to use? (The HMO probably will not pay for your treatment at hospitals that do not charge the HMO a lower price for your care.)
7. If I decide to be treated by a professional that is not a member of the HMO, will the HMO pay a portion of his or her bill?
8. Will the HMO pay part or all of the bill if I am away on vacation and cannot use an HMO provider?
9. Do you offer any programs to help prevent health problems such as premature birth, heart or lung disease, drug abuse, etc.? (Depending on your needs.)
10. How much will I be required to pay for:
    a. my monthly fee to belong to the HMO?
    b. prescription drugs?
    c. eyeglasses and contact lenses?
    d. time in a nursing home?
    e. visits to a mental health professional?
    f. dental care?
    g. visits to a physician?
    h. hospital room charges?
11. Are any changes in health care coverage planned or anticipated for members of this HMO?
12. Is nursing home care covered? For how long?
13. Is treatment for drug or alcohol dependence covered?
14. How much paperwork will I have to do to file a claim?
15. Are physical exams covered even if I don't have a problem?
16. Will treatment for a problem I had before enrolling in this insurance plan be covered?

17. Will I still be able to work with the caregivers that have treated me in the past?
18. What are the maximum benefits paid by this policy for each type of health care I might need?
19. Is this a "for-profit" HMO? Remember, HMO's that are out to make a profit have been shown to hospitalize their enrollees for shorter periods of time (Hillman, Pauly, & Kerstein, 1989). Some people believe that this suggests they are not giving certain customers enough care.
20. Are office visits for children free? (Your cost in belonging to an HMO or traditional insurance plan may largely depend on how many office visits your family is likely to make. With HMO's, these visits are usually free. Traditional insurance plans, however, may charge you a co-payment. If you have children who will need to make frequent office visits, you may do better financially by joining an HMO. This is because the extra attention your children require will be provided at no extra charge.)

Mental Health

If you will need mental health services there may be other questions for you to ask before signing up with any health insurance plan. Most of these questions listed below were borrowed from *The Common Sense Guide to Mental Health Care* (Ammer, 1982).

1. Is diagnostic consultation covered? If so, in the practitioner's office or only in the hospital? By a psychiatrist only or a psychologist or other mental health professional? Does it include psychological testing?
2. Is treatment for any nervous or mental disorder, regardless of previous illness, covered?
3. Are office visits to a social worker, psychiatrist, psychologist or other counselor covered? If so, how many are covered and is there any deductible?
4. Is electroconvulsive treatment ("shock therapy") covered in the hospital? In an outpatient setting?
5. Is hospitalization in a general hospital covered? In a

psychiatric hospital?
6. How long can the hospitalization last and be covered?
7. Is the cost of prescription drugs covered?
8. Is "partial hospitalization" (treatment at a hospital during the day) covered? What about day care, night care, half-way house?
9. Would an ambulance to the hospital or in a transfer situation be covered?
10. Is rehabilitation therapy covered?

Getting the Insurer to Pay

It should be clear by now that many employers go to great lengths to spend less on their employees' health insurance. One way many do this is to shop around and look at the prices of different plans, hoping to find the best value for their dollar. Then, they often choose the least expensive health insurance plans for their employees. Unfortunately, the quality of the health insurance may not be as important to them as low cost.

Because employers want to spend less, almost all insurers now keep close track of their customers' treatments. They do this to see whether or not the treatment being provided is necessary. This is referred to as "gate keeping." In many instances the "gatekeeper" is a nurse or a physician. The gatekeeper is an employee of the insurer, such as an HMO or traditional fee-for-service insurance company. If their decision is that treatment is not needed, the insurer will probably refuse to pay for the care.

For example, if you had heart problems your physician might advise you to have surgery. He or she could tell you that the operation is necessary and without it you could die. Your physician would then inform the insurance company of that opinion. At this point the gatekeeper would make a decision about whether or not the surgery was actually necessary. If the gatekeeper decided you could do without it, they might refuse to pay for the operation. They also might deny payment if they thought the treatment was "experimental." Quite a few insurance companies, for example, have refused to pay for temporary mechanical hearts, many of which are just being developed.

It is frustrating that not only does the insurance company try to take away the caregiver's ability to provide certain types of treatment, but it also limits consumers' freedom of choice. Rather than putting the control in your hands, the gatekeeper often makes the decision about the treatment you will receive.

In all fairness to insurance companies though, gate keeping probably has helped some consumers. This is because while they are gate keeping the insurance companies often keep detailed records about the successes and failures of different caregivers. This makes it possible for them to see when a particular professional's customers don't do well after treatment. It also helps them find those practitioners who perform too many tests or treat people too frequently. When this occurs, insurance companies often contact individual practitioners to say that a problem may exist. It is then up to the caregiver to see if the treatment he or she provides can be changed or improved.

If your insurance company refuses to pay for health care you believe is necessary, ask them to reconsider. There are procedures already in place to appeal such decisions that your insurer can help you follow. In fact, many insurance policies require you to first submit your complaint in writing to an arbitrator in the insurance company before you take other actions such as filing a lawsuit. At this point the insurance company may want to have another gatekeeper involved to offer a second opinion on whether or not you need the care. They may also want to talk with your caregiver or with you to learn more about why the treatment may be needed.

If arbitration fails, you can contact your state insurance commissioner. It is this official's responsibility to investigate consumers' grievances about insurance companies and to enforce any relevant laws that pertain to those complaints. Your insurance commissioner may also be an excellent source of information about such things as what types of treatment the insurance company is required to pay for, how long it is allowed to wait before paying your bills, and which caregivers the insurance company must allow you to visit.

If these efforts don't work, you may have to resort to other, more aggressive, tactics. You may even want to hold the insurance company responsible for the consequences of their decisions by threatening a lawsuit. One way to prepare for court is to ask your practitioner to write a letter about your treatment. This letter is to be copied and mailed to your insurance company. Here is an example:

> *Dear Mr. Smith:*
>
> *As you know, I recently have treated you for serious problems resulting from your (describe disease). It is my judgment that further treatment is absolutely necessary. This would consist of (describe the proposed treatment). If this treatment is not provided to you, I am quite concerned that you may suffer a number of problems. These include (list the possible consequences of not receiving treatment).*
>
> *Your insurance company has informed me that they have decided not to pay for this treatment. In their judgment, this care is not necessary. As you know, there are also no funds available to allow us to provide your care at no charge. As a result of the insurance company's decision and the lack of other sources of money to pay for your care, I predict that the needed treatment will not be made available to you.*
>
> *I will continue to do my best to treat you within the severe restrictions your insurance company has imposed. However, I cannot be held responsible for the consequences of their decision to refuse payment for your medically necessary treatment.*
>
> *Sincerely,*
> *Your Health Care Professional*
>
> *cc: Smith, Smith, and Smith Attorneys at Law*
> *910 Central Square Building Metropolis, USA.*

Notice that a copy of the letter has been sent to the biggest, meanest, most ferocious law firm in town. Your letter should probably be sent to a firm specializing in contract law or at least one that has a great deal of experience in that area. As distasteful as it may be to you, this intimidation may be effective and, in fact, necessary.

Medicaid And Medicare

There are two health insurance plans that are run by the federal government. The first of these, Medicaid, is for people who are disabled or have low incomes. One problem with this insurance is that it usually pays caregivers much less than they normally charge. In most cases the caregivers are forbidden from collecting the rest of their customary fees from the person they treat. As a result, many practitioners refuse to see people with this type of insurance.

Another federal insurance program is Medicare, which is designed for both the elderly and for anyone who is permanently disabled by kidney failure. As with Medicaid, there are drawbacks. People on Medicare have to pay for their own medications, they have to have all their treatments deemed "medically necessary," and there are many deductibles. In addition, most caregivers charge more than the maximum amount allowed by Medicare. When this happens, the consumer is usually responsible for paying the rest of the bill. Consumer Reports magazine (June 1989) found that this additional cost averaged 37 percent more than the basic "allowable" charge in 1988. In other words, it was common for consumers to have to pay more than a third of their own medical bills, even with Medicare coverage. Clearly, people with Medicare as their sole insurance plan are taking a chance of being saddled with many health care expenses. Often consumers wisely decide to buy more insurance to pay for the services not covered by Medicare.

Minorities and the elderly, two groups who commonly have Medicare and Medicaid insurance, sometimes have trouble receiving high quality health care in the hospital. This is because these insurance plans encourage caregivers in the hospital to provide as little treatment as possible. This is done by paying caregivers a set fee for treating an illness, no matter how long someone is in the hospital and no matter what treatment the hospital provides. In other words, if you are hospitalized, the insurance company may send the hospital one check, say for $3000. The hospital will get $3000 whether they send you home one day or one year later. Under this system, the less the hospital spends on you the greater their profits.

Consequently, many hospitals are reducing their own costs by doing things like sending ill people home earlier, performing fewer medical tests, and buying less expensive equipment. Physicians and other caregivers may be pressured to do only what is absolutely necessary. In fact, I remember one hospital administrator's comment that the general guideline in many hospitals is to do as little as possible for these consumers.

For example, an elderly hospitalized person in chronic pain might benefit from meetings with a physical therapist to learn relaxation and pain control techniques. Physical therapists, though, are often employees of hospitals. This means that the hospital pays their salary and, when possible, collects money from consumers for the treatment they provide. With Medicare and Medicaid, the hospital will probably not be able to collect more insurance money for the physical therapist's services. Because of this, the hospital may discourage them from treating this elderly person. Although the physical therapist's visits might make the person much more comfortable, his or her services are not essential for survival and would cost the hospital money.

Just like an HMO then, hospitals are often encouraged to cut costs. To the consumer this can mean poorer service. Some may be discharged from the hospital too early. Others find that they are discouraged from having medical tests performed that would give them an extra measure of safety. In any event, there is the potential for the quality of care they receive to suffer.

All of these problems make it important for people to be informed consumers who are willing to demand the care they need. They can't just assume their caregivers will spare no expense to give them the best possible treatment. The realities of today are that if you are on one of these insurance plans you need to know about your illness and the treatment you should be receiving. If you think you need to see a physical therapist, demand to see a physical therapist. If you want a second opinion from an experienced caregiver, insist that it be provided. And, if the hospital is reluctant, understand why, but don't let their hesitation prevent you from getting the best care our modern technology has to offer.

If You Become Disabled

If you are injured and unable to work, you may have an insurance plan that is responsible for paying medical bills, living expenses, or other costs resulting from your disability. Quite frequently when people are injured as a result of a job, they are entitled to insurance benefits as specified under "workers' compensation" laws. This insurance may be purchased by your employer. Workers' compensation benefits may pay you for part of your lost wages as well as the costs of needed medical treatments and rehabilitation. If you die as a result of your job, your dependents may also be entitled to other benefits. Not surprisingly, these costs can be very high, especially if you are out of work for a long time or need extended care. Because insurers don't want to be responsible for these bills, they have developed a number of strategies to avoid paying for your expenses.

Consider Felicia, a woman in her forties who suffered a back injury after slipping on a greasy floor at work. Because of her injury she will be unable to lift anything weighing over ten pounds for the rest of her life. She will also be in constant pain, with no hope for recovery. Felicia makes frequent visits to physicians, physical therapists, acupuncturists, and other expensive practitioners who are able to keep her more comfortable than she would be with no care at all. Further employment is probably out of the question, as most employers wouldn't want to take the risk of hiring her and having her develop more physical problems in her new job. So, as a result of her injury, she not only faces the prospect of lifelong pain, but she also needs to rely on others to help her with living expenses.

Felicia's insurance company certainly did not want to pay her expenses which could have eventually totaled hundreds of thousands of dollars. Predictably, they used a number of tactics to avoid incurring these costs. They first delayed payment of her medical bills, saying they would have to review all treatment to be certain it had been necessary. During the first few months after her injury, Felicia had received thousands of dollars in bills. She was legally responsible for paying them, even if her insurance company still had them under review. Since she was unemployed, she had no hope of paying even a small portion of her expenses. The insurance company also refused to pay for her rent, as her contract clearly required them to do. This went on for six months and she was soon forced to move in with relatives, sell many of her possessions, and go deeply into debt.

The insurance company's next move was to send her to a practitioner of their choice to see whether or not she was actually able to go back to work. This caregiver's decision, which was much different from the opinions of all her earlier professionals, was that she could be employed. Further, the caregiver said that there was no medical reason she should be feeling as much pain as she reported. The insurance company, upon receiving his report, offered to pay off her past debts but refused to pay for any future medical care or living expenses.

At this point Felicia finally went to an experienced attorney. She learned from him that the insurance company's strategy was to put her in a financially desperate situation where she would be willing to accept any settlement they offered. They did this by delaying payment for her expenses and sending her to one of their own "hired gun" caregivers who they knew would help them justify not paying her bills. Luckily, her attorney was able to intervene just in time. With his help she forced the insurance company to pay all of her past and future medical bills as well as give her $25,000 for living expenses. In addition to seeing an attorney, Felicia might have filed a complaint with the insurance commissioner in her state. She knew that there were state laws that prevented insurance companies from postponing payment of her bills for such a long time.

It's ironic that insurance companies' attempts to save cash frequently backfire and end up costing them more money. They also can create a lot of suffering for consumers. This often happens when insurers refuse to pay for necessary health care. Sooner or later problems occur that would have been avoided if the consumer had received proper treatment originally.

Roger, a man in his late fifties, experienced these problems with his insurance carrier after he had been knocked unconscious in an automobile accident. A few months after his injury he returned to his job as a foreman for a construction company. Once back to work he noticed that he had trouble remembering employees' names, the correct construction materials to order, and when to mail payroll checks. He also learned that he could no longer understand blueprints and experienced a tremendous amount of fatigue after only a few hours on the job.

When he could tolerate these symptoms no longer, he went to a number of caregivers for help. The people he saw decided that he had suffered brain damage during the car accident. They suggested that he enter a local rehabilitation program designed to help treat his difficulties thinking clearly and with fatigue. The program they recommended was quite expensive. Predictably, his insurance company refused to pay for the program. They said that one of their professionals found little evidence of brain damage and thought he probably was exaggerating his symptoms in order to avoid work.

In reality, his brain damage was causing him to make serious mistakes that needlessly endangered both him and his employees. On several occasions he forgot to use a safety belt when walking on steel girders ten stories above ground. He also insisted that his employees work outside even though ice that had formed on the building made that hazardous. The owner of the company became concerned about these safety problems and about the construction which was falling far behind schedule.

After a few months, Roger lost his job and had serious financial problems. Although he found two more jobs, he lost each of them in a few weeks because of his poor judgment and memory. Understandably, he became quite depressed and needed many expensive counseling sessions. To their dismay, the insurance company was forced to pay for these meetings as well as for some of his living expenses.

Two years after his injury the insurance company finally

decided to pay for the rehabilitation program that originally had been recommended. They thought that it would be worth the expense if it helped him return to work. Their hope was that if he could hold a job he would support himself and not need further counseling. They were also persuaded by Roger's new attorney, who aggressively fought for the care he needed. After completing the program, Roger was able to hold down a part time job and pay most of his own bills. His self-esteem returned and he didn't need the mental health services that he had relied on in the past.

It's clear that if the insurance company had originally paid for the expensive treatment program it would have avoided having to pay for many of his living expenses and counseling sessions. The insurance company's refusal to pay for treatment caused Roger to suffer both emotionally and financially. It also eventually cost the insurance company more money.

A good source for further information is the book *Choosing the Right Health Care Plan* by Henry Berman M.D. and Louisa Rose. It is can be ordered from Consumer Reports Books, 9180 LeSaint Drive, Fairfield, OH 45014-5452.

CHAPTER 4

Keeping On Top of Your Care

"Everything is all right. The great and powerful OZ has got matters well in hand, I hope."
*–Professor Marvel, (***The Wizard of OZ,** *1939)*

Why Learn About It Yourself?

Some people look to one or two caregivers for all of their health care information. They don't read about their illnesses in libraries or even get second opinions. This is often because they are scared by technical articles or are afraid of making their practitioners mad. But more knowledgeable consumers usually can find and understand information written about their care. They also feel free to ask for second opinions. These skills are important because caregivers often don't tell people enough about their illnesses to make it possible for them to be informed consumers.

Sometimes it's really astounding how little people know about their own illnesses. In one study of 200 people with cancer (Cassileth, Zupkis, Sutton-Smith, & March, 1980) only 60% were able to correctly describe the treatments that were recommended by their physicians. Only 41% could name one major risk of therapy and a mere 27% could name one alternative form of treatment. Another study of women who were eventually treated with radiation therapy for breast cancer showed that over half were first incorrectly told that there was no alternative to having their breast removed. One caregiver even discouraged a woman from having radiation therapy instead of surgery by incorrectly stating that it would "make your breast look and feel like a dried, old apple" (Greiner & Weiler, 1983).

Even when they ask, consumers often have difficulty getting the information they need to make educated decisions about their own treatments. Consider, for example, the plight of a 34 year-old woman who was just told that she would need a mastectomy to treat her breast cancer.

> *...I managed to keep my wits about me and asked for literature on the subject [mastectomy]. All they could find on the ward was a Mastectomy Association leaflet produced some eight years previously and bearing the association's old address and telephone number. It... was illustrated with color photographs of pleasant elderly ladies pruning roses and some slightly younger ones pushing prostheses into sagging beige nylon bras. (Prior, 1987).*

Exactly what decisions, you may ask, can I make when I'm ill? Warner Slack M.D., from Harvard Medical School, has addressed this question in his article on "patient power" (Slack, 1972). He first discusses moral decisions that consumers face when they are ill. Moral decisions are based on consumers' personal preferences and wishes. These include such things as someone's willingness to tolerate discomfort after surgery in order to increase the chances of survival. In other words, some consumers make personal decisions to have surgery because they believe that the possible benefits are worth the pain. Dr. Slack makes the important point that the consumer will not necessarily make the same moral decision that the caregiver would if the practitioner were confronted with the same illness.

It is here that he notes there is the potential for conflict. Many caregivers have been accustomed to caring for people as they would wish to be cared for themselves. In so doing they may impose their own values upon decisions made in behalf of their customers. Here, a caregiver may encourage a person to have surgery, submit to a painful test, or receive a certain treatment because the caregiver thinks that the benefits would be worth the pain. Dr. Slack believes that consumers should be the ones to make these choices. It is they who may have to go into debt, suffer discomfort, or risk being injured by the treatment.

It is his position that the professional should describe the possible outcomes of tests or treatments and then let the consumer decide which, if any, will be done. Of course, it's essential for the consumer to get all of the information needed to make these decisions. This might include information on the likelihood of discovering medical problems or causing pain, incapacitation, death, or financial burden if the consumer chooses to submit to the procedure. Similarly, the pros and cons of not going through with the procedure should be described.

In order to make value judgments, people are often forced to turn to libraries or other experts for information on health care. This happens for at least three reasons. First, caregivers often are not willing to spend enough time with people to give them the information they need. There are frequently shortages of health care professionals and their time may be limited. Second, the caregivers may deliberately withhold information in order to increase their power over consumers. After all, if their customers don't know much about their own problems they won't be able to challenge what caregivers recommend. Lastly, it is often impossible for one caregiver to know everything about the treatment of an illness. Many practitioners, with different types of professional training and specialty areas, may be needed to present all the treatment options.

Dr. Slack recommends that while consumers should be in charge of moral choices, the physician should make medical decisions. Presumably, these would often involve such technical matters as which medication to prescribe, the timing of surgery, and so forth. This frequently makes sense, as most caregivers are much more skilled in making these sorts of choices than untrained laymen. The professionals are the ones who are often in the best position to recommend the most effective therapy or prescribe the medication with the fewest dangerous side effects.

The problem, though, is that caregivers sometimes make mistakes. One recent study (Lesar & Pohl, 1990) of physicians in teaching hospitals showed that physicians made almost two and one-half errors each day when prescribing drugs. Over half of these mistakes were serious enough to be health risks. Because of these sorts of problems, many people understandably are uncomfortable leaving all the decisions, even technical ones, up to their caregivers. Instead, these consumers decide to learn as much as possible about their own health care. They hope to make some of their own decisions and be certain they are getting the best treatment available.

This is not to suggest that consumers should ignore their caregiver's recommendations. A professional's advice should usually be respected. However, almost everything a consumer is told should be confirmed. Usually this is done either by a second opinion from another practitioner or with written materials.

Many people have talked about the "luxury of being a patient." This refers to the belief that when people are ill they should be able to count on others to make decisions about their care. The reasoning is often that people need to spend their energy "just getting well" and shouldn't be bothered with the burden of making decisions. Further, it is often quite stressful for people to make decisions at times when they may already be both physically and emotionally spent. In fact, even caregivers sometimes appropriately chastise other professionals for encouraging a consumer to make too many choices at these difficult times.

Even I would agree that some people should take a less active role in their own care. Some are so sick that they don't have the energy to study their own illnesses. Others are confused because medications interfere with their thinking and some aren't smart enough to understand their care. For these few people the best decision often is to let others take over. This is probably more often a good choice when understanding technical matters than when making moral decisions. Even very sick people who don't know much about health care can almost always tell what they want; they just can't make good use of the more complicated technical information.

These instances, though, are the exception rather than the rule. Most of the time people can improve the quality of their care by helping to make decisions about their own treatments. But one price they may pay for better service is increased anxiety. It can be scary to know about your illness. And it's even more frightening to many people to learn how to make decisions about their own treatments. In order to avoid having this anxiety, many people actually look for caregivers who won't tell them very much. Instead, they prefer to "follow orders" and not ask questions. I remember one woman whose practitioner told her next to nothing about her treatment. She was happy to take advantage of the "luxury of being a patient." When he left town to practice somewhere else she found herself with a caregiver who explained nearly every detail of her care. After her first visit she left his office in a panic. She described him as a "terrible man" who "didn't know anything about working with patients."

Knowing about your own health care may raise your anxiety but it should not stop you from learning about your condition and pushing for high quality service. Consider your anxiety to be just be one more thing you have to endure to insure that you are treated competently. In fact, some people (e.g., Janis, 1958) think some anxiety can actually be beneficial. It may motivate people to prepare for things like athletic competitions, classroom tests, and yes, even medical procedures. It's only when this anxiety reaches extreme levels that it interferes with attempts to cope.

Using the Library

The library is one of your best sources of health care information. It often plays an essential role in helping consumers make educated decisions about their own treatments. Libraries not only make a great deal of information available to you, but they are easier to use than they were years ago. Many people remember the drudgery of paging through hundreds of little white index cards to find a book. If they were lucky they found what they wanted but then had to wait several weeks for the book to be returned by someone else. Today the computer has revolutionized the library and made it much easier to get information about almost any topic related to health care.

Fortunately, most hospitals and medical schools have specialized "medical libraries" that hold much reading material. These libraries can usually be used by anyone in the community. The librarians at medical libraries are also often quite skilled in helping people locate information on health care. If a medical library is nearby, it might save you time to begin your search for information there.

If there is no medical library in your area, don't give up. You may still be able to find what you need using university or public libraries. Although the librarians in these facilities may not be experienced in locating information on health care, they still might be a great help in your search for useful material that you can understand.

These days there are many books and articles written for the layperson, who has absolutely no training in health care. Many of these easy-to-understand materials are listed in a publication called the *Consumer Health and Nutrition Index* (Orynx Press), which you may find at your library. (Complete references for all publications are included in the reference section near the end of this book.) This index lists current articles from 86 periodicals published by centers around the country such as Harvard Medical School and the Mayo Clinic. It also includes articles from magazines like *Consumer Reports*, *Cosmopolitan*, and *Family Circle*. Again, all of the articles are written for the person with little or no health care training.

Good Housekeeping has published *The New Good Housekeeping Family Health And Medical Guide* (editor, 1989). this includes five chapters with information on such subjects as medical tests, breast-feeding, drug abuse, and disorders of aging. For more specific information on medical testing you may want to locate a copy of *Instructions for Patients: Medical Tests and Diagnostic Procedures* (Griffith, 1989). This book presents information in easy-to-understand tables that can be photocopied. It explains such things as the purpose of the test, the risks of being tested, and how being given the test will feel.

Mental health problems and treatments are described in *The Family Mental Health Encyclopedia* (Bruno, 1989). This book outlines the use of various drugs and therapies used to treat mental disorders. It also offers descriptions of the different specialties of mental health professionals.

If you are having surgery the book *General Surgery* (Pratt & Sarewitz, 1988) may give you a good idea of what to expect. One of the outstanding features of this book is it's clear and simple illustrations of the surgical procedures. It also discusses why surgery is performed, it's risks and benefits, and it's possible complications.

Complete Guide to Symptoms, Illness & Surgery (Griffith, 1989) is written for the layperson who wants to learn more about the possible meanings of physical symptoms or who needs other general information about illnesses. This might be an especially useful source for those wishing to double check on their own diagnosis and treatment. Here, the consumer could first look up a symptom, such as abdominal pain, and learn that it could be caused by such problems as kidney stones, infection, or heart attack. They could then go to a different section of the book to find information about the problem as well as learn about appropriate treatments and possible complications.

Those wanting to know more about medication can turn to *The Essential Guide to Prescription Drugs* (Long, 1992). One way you can use this book is to first look up your illness. After reading a thorough description of the disorder, you will see a list of drugs that are used to treat that illness. The goals of drug treatment, as well as the chances of recovery, by using medication are explained. Another section lists individual medications and describes how they work, the usual dosages, the risks and benefits from taking the drug, and how you can know if you should not be taking the medication.

The Physician's Desk Reference (1993) is an annual publication written primarily for health care professionals wishing to know about medications. Although it is written in technical language, it gives complete information about almost all prescription drugs approved for use in the United States. It is a widely available book that can be found in almost every medical office and hospital ward. So, if you are ever at one of these places and need information about medications quickly, it should be easy to ask to see a copy of the *Physician's Desk Reference*. Also, because there are health care professionals nearby you should be able to find someone to help you understand the more technical material it contains.

For more information about those impressive sounding medical terms (such as "abetalipoproteinemia" and "ablepharous") you can turn to *Melloni's Illustrated Medical Dictionary* (Melloni,

1985). It's organized much like an ordinary dictionary with easily understandable definitions for unfamiliar words. It also has well done illustrations of many parts of the body.

Finally, many people will want to locate health or medical organizations. *The Encyclopedia of Associations* (Koek, Martin, & Novallo, 1993) can help you locate thousands of organizations throughout the world, many of which could provide you with health care information. It contains a brief description of organizations such as the National Institute of Mental Health along with their addresses and telephone numbers. A consumer who wishes to learn more about a particular disorder may be able to receive that information by contacting the appropriate agency.

These are just a few of the hundreds of publications written for the layperson that can help you learn more about health care. Your librarian should be able to help you find many more books and articles on almost any health-related subject. Probably the major limitation of this literature is that it might not include information on health problems that require rare or new treatments. Highly specialized surgery, newly developed medications, or other uncommonly used physical and psychological therapies are usually first reported in more technical articles primarily written for professionals. Usually these treatments are described in the books and articles printed for the general public only after they have been used for some time. It is in these cases that you may have to turn to the this more technical literature to find out about your illness.

Perhaps one of the easiest ways to find this technical material is with a "computer search." With this service, a librarian uses a computer to look through thousands of scientific articles or books to find information on a particular subject. Imagine that you needed to know about a new type of eye surgery. To do a computer search, the librarian would first connect his or her computer to a larger "database" over the telephone line. The database may be in another computer, perhaps in a different city, that contains the titles, authors, and one paragraph summaries (called "abstracts") of the scientific articles written on that eye surgery. The librarian would then have his or her computer select those articles that would be of most help to you and have their titles, abstracts, and other reference information printed out on paper for you to keep. It may be especially helpful for the librarian to provide you with the abstracts of each journal article, since they describe the main points of the paper. It usually costs a bit more to do this, but you'll probably find the extra information is worth the expense.

After you have read about the articles selected by the computer, you can choose those that you think would be most useful. They might be in your library, especially if it has many journals or books on health care. But if your library doesn't have these journals or books, the librarian will probably order them. This will mean you will have to wait a few days or weeks. The important thing to remember though is today no matter where you live, your librarian can probably get the health care information you need.

Even if you don't live near a library with a computer, your librarian can direct you to one that does. And, if you can't travel there yourself, you should be able to arrange for the computer search with the help of your local librarian. Your librarian will ask you about the information you need and probably also ask for payment in advance. He or she will then contact another library that can carry out a computer search and tell them about the information you are requesting. That second library should then send the computer print-out to you in the mail within a few days.

If there is no library in your area, you can call a library yourself to request a computer search. Although this probably isn't standard procedure, there is no technical reason why you would need to be present for a computer search. Understandably, the librarian may ask you to send payment in advance to pay for the computer search and postage. After you receive the computer print-out, you can circle those materials that you want to read. Then mail the print-out back to the librarian (along with a large stamped mailing envelope with your return address) and ask for a photocopy of the articles you requested and that they be returned to you in the mail.

If you order a computer search over the telephone, be sure to ask the librarian to include the articles' abstracts. This is especially important if you don't live close to a library where you can quickly skim the articles themselves. The difficulty is that you may not be able to understand the material from the titles alone.

You could therefore find that the abstracts are essential to help you understand the articles' main points.

Computer searches are a fantastic time saver; they search through libraries of information in seconds. Depending on how many articles or books you request you might pay somewhere between $15 to $45 for this service. If possible, have a librarian assist you who is experienced in helping people find out about health care. These more knowledgeable librarians not only are often much more skilled in performing the computer searches, but they might also be able to suggest reading material. In addition, these experienced librarians might recognize the "big name" professionals in your area who have published or have the most expertise. While certainly not guaranteeing competence, these qualifications usually assure you that a practitioner has had a certain degree of experience. If he or she has published articles or books on your illness, it also means that person's work has probably been praised by his or her colleagues.

There are exceptions to this however. In your library search you will notice that most scientific articles are written by more than one person. In almost all cases each of these people did not contribute equally to conducting the research and writing the article. It is customary for those who have contributed the most to the project to be listed near the beginning of this list of authors, usually located on the first page of the article. The others, who have made less of a contribution, typically have their names added on near the end of the list. As with many group projects though, one person may have done most of the work, the next might not have done anything, and the last may have tried to get all the credit. If this sort of thing did happen, the one who was listed first may not have been the one who did the most work or knew the most about the study.

Sometimes, authors with their names near the end have not helped at all in carrying out the study or writing the article. In fact, they may never even have heard of the project until after it was published. This is often the case in the medical field where caregivers with power or prestige have their names added to the article as a professional courtesy. This might include the head of the hospital or university department in which the study was performed.

An alternative to going to the library for health care information is to call the staff of Planetree at (415) 923-3680. Planetree is an organization created, in part, to provide people with information about their health care. For a reasonable fee, they will mail you an in-depth packet of information on your health problem.

The National Health Information Clearinghouse may also be able to provide you with information on your medical condition. They might be especially helpful if you are trying to get in touch with an organization created to help people with a specific illness or even a rare disease. This organization can be reached at (800) 336-4797.

Understanding Articles on Health Care

It's difficult for most people to understand scientific articles on health care. This is because they are usually written in technical language for professionals who have had years of experience. So, if you need to turn to this literature, don't be surprised if at first little or none of it makes much sense.

To understand technical articles, don't be shy about asking others to explain important points. Perhaps you could study each of the articles before your appointment with your practitioner. Then, during your appointment you could ask that professional to explain the things that you don't understand. Remember, an important part of your caregiver's job is to help you know about your illness and treatment. You shouldn't worry about asking for extra time so your practitioner can explain the articles you found.

Next, read the articles again and again. Have both a medical dictionary and a Webster's handy for words you don't understand. Don't give up after reading the articles just two or three times. Expect that it will take you a lot of effort to understand the material thoroughly.

Be sure to read as many articles on your illness as you can. This is important because the experts often disagree and give conflicting opinions in different articles. You want to see how much the experts are in agreement on the diagnosis and treatment of your illness. If the authors all seem to say the same thing and their recommendations are consistent with those of your caregiver, you are probably getting good advice. In this case you may have to make few decisions about the best treatment. If, however, you notice that each author seems to endorse a different way of diagnosing or treating an illness, your task will probably be more difficult. You may need to give careful consideration to each viewpoint. Your practitioner might be especially helpful in explaining the pros and cons of each of the opinions you have read.

When reading scientific studies on health care, you will probably notice that many articles describe research that was done with hundreds of people. The authors of these studies will often make statements such as "this form of therapy was found to help 75 percent of the persons who were treated" or "just over 20 percent of those who received this therapy suffered from side effects...." Researchers often study many people because this makes it possible for them to get precise statistics like these. The research projects are designed to see exactly how effective, dangerous, or useful a procedure will be in the future.

Working with so many people gives these researchers a great deal of useful information. This information is usually much more reliable than most people's beliefs, which are based on their own observations of fewer people. For a practical example, imagine that you have just been diagnosed as having the same type of cancer that three of your friends have had in the past. Two of your friends have died and one is still living. You remember that the two who are no longer living both received a cancer treatment called "medication A." The other friend, who is still alive and doing well, was given a totally different pill called "medication B." Because the two people on medication A died, you have decided that you want to get medication B, which seems to be more effective. Yet, when reading a research study where these two treatments were used in 500 people, you learn that people given medication B only rarely recover from their cancer. Furthermore, the study showed that 90 percent of people given medication A survived their disease.

Your difficult choice at this point is to decide what to believe:

your personal experience with three of your friends, or the scientific study of five hundred people. It's surprising how many people would dismiss the research findings and choose to take the medication that helped their two friends. What they don't appreciate is that their friends probably died taking medication A and lived taking medication B due to chance. Even though your personal observations suggest otherwise, the scientific study shows that overall people have a 90 percent chance of survival if they take medication A. Logically, it would be a mistake to choose the medication that seemed to help your friends.

One writer (Cassileth 1989) has remarked that even some surgeons have made these kinds of mistakes. Several years ago it was shown that in some people with breast cancer removal of only the cancerous lump and radiation therapy was just as effective as total mastectomy. Some surgeons dismissed these results, holding to their long-standing belief of the greater chance of a cure with removal of the breast. In other words, though they were confronted with the results of an international study of many people, they still based decisions on their own more limited experience.

Also, your reading might make it clear that there is more than one way to treat your problem. Each article, book, or newsletter, in fact, might advocate a totally different approach. Not only may this make your selection of treatments much more difficult, but it may raise your anxiety because there is no clear cut choice for you to make. This should remind you how difficult your caregivers' jobs often become. They frequently have to make very difficult judgment calls about which treatment to recommend when no single treatment is definitely superior to another.

Teaching Your Provider

After your studies, you may actually be more knowledgeable than your caregivers about your disease. Many people with a fairly rare illness called "myasthenia gravis," for example, are afraid of going into the hospital because they think their caregivers will know less about treating their problems than they do (Sneddon, 1980). Some of these people even worry that if they were hospitalized their medications would be taken away by inept practitioners. They know that withholding medication could cause serious physical problems, including death. Some of these people will even resort to hiding pills to stay in control of their own care (Sneddon, 1980).

To prevent these sorts of problems, you may need to educate your caregiver. One way to do this is to give your practitioner some written information on your disease. A copy of an article or one brief chapter out of a book might be read quickly and have much information. It's also usually not as threatening for caregivers to find information in these written sources as it is to learn it from customers. Another advantage is that written materials may help establish your credibility and let others know that you plan to work with them while you are treated.

You could suggest that the article or chapter be included in your medical chart. This may be an especially good idea if you are being treated in a hospital or clinic by many caregivers. This way all of your practitioners will be able to read the material as they look through your records.

Being a good teacher may be especially important in emergencies. One way to let others know basic information about your disease and treatment is to have it engraved on a medical bracelet or necklace. These are available at the prescription counters of most drug stores. Thus, if you can't talk in an emergency you can still inform others of your disease and describe the proper treatment.

You can even order a special "Medic Alert®" bracelet from Medic Alert, Turlock, California, 95381-1009. The names of your medical conditions are engraved on this bracelet along with the telephone number of a 24-hour information line. If you need emergency care, your provider simply calls the long distance number to receive more details about your condition. If you would like to order one of these bracelets, call 1-800-ID ALERT.

Another option is to carry a detailed written description of your illness in your wallet or purse. This could easily include several pages of information. It may be a good practice to engrave on your bracelet or necklace instructions on where to find this more detailed information. For example, "myasthenia gravis patient, see card in wallet for instructions on emergency treatment" might help emergency personnel learn about your illness more quickly. If you do this, be sure to have your regular caregiver check the medical information you carry for accuracy and completeness.

Whenever you need to educate your caregivers try to appear as calm as possible. This will make you more believable and make it more likely that others will follow your advice. You may want to begin by describing your diagnosis and symptoms clearly. Tell what helps your symptoms and what makes them worse. You might also insist that your caregivers call professionals who have helped you in the past.

You don't want your wishes dismissed because your emotions stop you from calmly and effectively discussing your illness. I remember one young man named "Kevin" who had myasthenia gravis, a neurological disease that can cause sudden muscle weakness, paralysis, and even suffocation. One day he had a sudden attack of this illness. Soon after it began he was unable to move. Kevin could not communicate and was even having difficulty breathing.

Kevin's father, aunt and uncle were with him when he had his attack. None had been coached on the proper first aid to use in this situation. As he lay on the floor, his father panicked and screamed at him to try to stand up and move. Next, his aunt and uncle argued with each other about whether or not to call an ambulance. All the commotion made it very difficult for him to concentrate, something that he needed to do to help himself breathe.

Five minutes after his attack began, Kevin's relatives finally decided to call an ambulance. Once in the hospital, the emergency room team had no idea how to administer aid for this unusual problem. Again there was much yelling and confusion. He was given too much oxygen which caused him to breathe too quickly. The emergency room staff mistakenly thought he was breathing fast because of anxiety. To slow his breathing he was mistakenly given medication that could have killed him. Luckily, he survived and eventually regained his strength.

Understandably, Kevin was furious at his relatives and the

emergency room staff for his poor care. He had no choice but to make certain that if he had another serious attack, others would know how to treat him correctly. So, the next day he severely scolded his father for panicking. He also planned to write a scathing letter to several of the hospital administrators, naming the hospital staff who had mistreated him. What he didn't consider was that if he had another attack the same relatives would probably have to take him to that same emergency room. After being scolded, few of these people would probably feel like rolling out the red carpet. His anger may have interfered with his future medical treatment.

Instead of writing that nasty letter, Kevin decided to use more tact. He thought that it would be in his best interests to educate the other people about the proper care to administer should he have another emergency. To accomplish this, he first chose to write a letter to the hospital's "patient representative." This hospital employee investigates complaints and works in consumers' behalf to improve hospital care. This letter discussed, without naming names, his treatment in the emergency room and how his care there could have been improved. The letter did not sound blaming and was written in a rather "matter-of-fact" tone.

In addition to the letter, Kevin met with the emergency room team and gave them brochures and other information on how to treat someone with myasthenia gravis. He also showed them literature published by drug companies that showed how the medicine that they gave him in the emergency room could have resulted in his death. While at first quite defensive, the emergency room personnel eventually had to admit that their treatment had been wrong.

A few days later, he spoke with his family physician, who had learned of his emergency treatment and of his attempts to educate his caregivers. The physician explained that he was getting a reputation among the staff for being "too aggressive" by telling others how to provide medical care. He explained that the hospital staff never liked it when customers told them how to do their jobs.

Apparently even Kevin's best efforts to avoid humiliating his caregivers were not totally successful. He certainly couldn't have risked letting himself be hurt in the future because incompetent staff had a hard time taking advice. Kevin had no choice but to risk the emergency team's wrath in hopes of being treated correctly if the problem occurred again. This was a tradeoff. He accepted the fact that he might bruise some egos and create ill feelings in order to educate his health care professionals. The most that he could hope for was to try to keep the staff's anger at a minimum. He did this by acting in a calm and rational manner, providing them with written information about his disease, and not using their names to embarrass them in front of the patient representative.

So many people believe it's their duty to make practitioners feel better when they get upset. If a professional gets riled because of their decisions, they often think they should smooth things over and try to make amends, even if it means going along with a health care decision they don't like. Fortunately, Kevin didn't make this mistake. He knew that it wasn't his responsibility to soothe his caregivers when they got bent out of shape because of his assertiveness. That was not his problem, except, of course, if their anger might cause him to receive poorer care in the future.

Some people wisely decide to educate their caregivers or push for changes in their own treatments only when it's really necessary. In order to avoid being known as nags, they ignore some of their caregivers' less costly mistakes. As a result, caregivers may pay more attention when there is a legitimate concern about care. Kevin's complaints about his treatment for myasthenia gravis were clearly an example of important problems that needed to be discussed. If he had pestered his caregivers earlier about wanting minor changes in his medication, more frequent appointments with his practitioners, and so forth, his caregivers would probably have been even less likely to listen to his objections.

People like Kevin who try to talk tactfully but openly with their caregivers are certainly acting in their own best interests. Good practitioner-consumer communication has a number of benefits (Kaplan, Greenfield, & Ware, 1989). One obvious benefit is that it helps consumers and practitioners exchange important information. But there is much more. Being able to talk with a caregiver may be a great motivater. Respected caregivers may be able to encourage people to better care for themselves. Practitioners often do this by boosting people's self-confidence with "pep talks." Just being able to talk intelligently with a caregiver and having one's views respected improves many people's self-confidence. Good communication also makes it possible for people to get some emotional support that they might need so desperately. Not surprisingly, a number of studies already have shown that better physician-consumer communication often is associated with improved health (see Kaplan, Greenfield, & Ware, 1989).

By the way, patient representatives such as the one Kevin contacted can be found in most hospitals. They may be a great help if you have problems or complaints about your care that you can't work out quietly on your own. For example, some hospitals restrict customers' privileges to use the hospital library. In these cases the patient representatives are sometimes able to pull strings and make it possible for consumers to use the libraries to study about their illnesses. Perhaps you are afraid of being hurt by a medical test or treatment. If so, the patient representative might be able to reduce your risk or calm your worries. And, if you are shaken out of bed at 5:30 A.M. every morning to be weighed by a hospital orderly, the patient representative might also intervene.

Changing and Directing Your Treatment

There are many different ways consumers and caregivers view each other. One perspective, held by some consumers, is that practitioners should make all decisions about treatment. Many caregivers like this role. They enjoy making choices for others and dislike having their opinions questioned. Other consumers view caregivers as advisors and technicians. They think practitioners should give them the information they need to make decisions about their own health. In most cases, the caregiver also is seen as someone who is useful because of technical skills, such as knowing how to rebuild wasted muscles with special exercises. From this second perspective, the caregiver makes no decisions for the consumer, but instead advises the consumer about the pros and cons of different treatments. Obviously, it is this second perspective that I am encouraging the reader to adopt. It helps the customer to have a healthy skepticism, or an attitude of "buyer beware," that may be so important to protect his or her health.

It is interesting to see what happens in the relationships between consumers and caregivers after customers treat "doctor's orders" as merely suggestions. Some caregivers acknowledge a questioning attitude in passing and then continue with what they would have done anyway. When consumers disagree they may also say they aren't being cooperative and ask them instead to see another professional.

What these caregivers do is make the serious mistake of believing that they are in charge of treatment. Warner Slack M.D. (1977) has written at length that physicians, in general, should not believe that they are responsible for their customers' decisions about health care. Instead, he states, they should simply offer plans of action just like an electrician, an accountant, or any other vendor. They should leave it up to the consumer to decide what should be done.

Slack further argues that if caregivers give up the role of making all the decisions, consumers will be much more likely to follow their practitioners' advice. They will have greater self-esteem and feel as if they have more control. This also benefits the caregiver who would no longer be seen as solely responsible for the sometimes unfortunate consequences of treatment decisions.

Consumers can learn from physicians when it comes to taking control over their own treatment. It's a standard joke that when physicians are hospitalized they are seen as "bad patients" by hospital staff. Many staff dread having to take care of the physician who will insist that things are done in a particular way. They are known for constantly questioning decisions made in their behalf, giving orders to hospital workers, and letting everyone know if a mistake has been made. In part, this occurs because physicians know more about medical treatment than the typical consumer. They are in a better position to make educated decisions quickly about their own care. They usually don't have to run to the library to know if a blood test is necessary or if they should be having a special diet. Physicians have also earned this reputation because they are used to being in charge. It's usually very much out of character for them to let others choose treatments for them. In fact, letting someone else make their decisions can make them very anxious because it would mean they would no longer be in control over their own fate.

But these things don't make physicians "bad patients." Quite the opposite, in fact, is true. They may be among the most educated of consumers. They are also likely to get the highest quality care. The fact that they are sometimes irritating to hospital staff is beside the point. It is simply the price that is paid when they catch caregivers' mistakes and insist on receiving the best treatment. And as one physician commented, "...better bad than dead. Being a doctor may lower your risks in that most hazardous of places-the American hospital" (Felson, 1987)

Let's look at some of the situations in which consumers are likely to disagree with their diagnoses or treatments (see Haug & Lavin, 1983). First, the articles or books you have read may contradict the advice given by your caregiver. Your reading material may suggest a different diagnosis or treatment. It may even describe some risks that your caregiver did not discuss with you. When this happens, be sure to talk about your reservations with your practitioner. In fact, it might be a good idea to let your caregiver read the materials that disagree with his or her point of view. This is especially important if you are suffering from a problem that your professional rarely encounters. In this case you may actually be able to help your caregiver learn about the most appropriate and current treatments.

It is important to remember that no article or book can give good advice about your individual treatment. Written materials cannot take into consideration all the special problems (such as allergies, etc.) that might prevent you from being treated in a certain way. Your health care professional can help you with these issues and tell you why the best treatment for you may be different from those described in your reading material.

You may also have received second or third opinions that contradict your caregiver. In this case you may want to arrange a conference, where all your providers meet in the same room to talk about your treatment. This is often helpful in a busy hospital where your caregivers may communicate with each other only by writing notes in your chart. Many people may be involved in your care without ever talking directly to each other. This usually results in very poor communication between practitioners who really should know a lot about the other caregivers' opinions.

You may think that your health care practitioner has not examined you thoroughly enough or performed the necessary tests. This could be enough reason to have less confidence in his or her judgment. It could also present you with an especially difficult situation if she recommends radical or dangerous treatments such as surgery on the basis of an insufficient examination. These are the times when you may want to put off treatment or insist on another evaluation by a more thorough professional.

You may be concerned that the treatment is not needed or is too drastic. This might occur if someone with a very mild depression was told to enter the hospital for treatment. In addition to the unnecessary expense, such a decision might be harmful to the consumer who may have to take a break from work. Not only would this result in a loss of income but probably self-esteem as well, something already in short supply in many depressed people. Similarly, if surgery is recommended by only one caregiver another consumer may want to postpone treatment until everyone is certain that it is necessary.

On the other hand, you may think that your treatment isn't aggressive enough. For example, some women with breast cancer have chosen to have an entire breast removed instead of just the cancerous lumps. This is because in their case a total mastectomy was more likely to result in a complete cure of their cancer. Removal of just the lump might be easier for them to accept psychologically, but may not be as likely to cure their disease. They insisted that their breasts be removed for what they believed was a higher likelihood of recovery.

Your caregiver may suggest a treatment that you think will not work or could be harmful. Clearly, this is a good reason to question the safety and effectiveness of the therapy that is recommended. You may also decide to talk with other caregivers at this point.

This would help you find out more about the treatment your health care practitioner suggested and to see if there are better or safer treatments available.

You may disagree with your health care professional if he or she doesn't believe your description of your symptoms. Your caregiver may see you as a chronic complainer or as someone who tends to exaggerate the severity of health problems. A professional may even chalk your problems up as "psychological" and not give them the attention or treatment they deserve. While there are many complainers and people who exaggerate, you don't want your illness to be ignored because someone thinks you can't report your symptoms accurately.

Sometimes you may need to be quite forceful and move quickly when challenging a health care provider's treatment. I remember one young man, Ron, who was hospitalized for an inflammation of his colon called "ulcerative colitis." He was in very serious condition where he couldn't even eat. Ron's physician, a highly skilled caregiver, suggested that he first take medication to see if it helped his condition. The plan was to remove Ron's colon if the medication didn't work in three or four days. It was important to perform this surgery on schedule if the medicine did not stop the inflammation. This was because if his condition did not improve a hole could develop in his inflamed colon. Any perforation might cause serious infection and possibly result in his death.

After a few days in the hospital it was clear that the drugs weren't working and that Ron would need surgery. Unfortunately though, after his third day in the hospital his physician left the state for a three day conference. In the physician's absence were several new physicians who took over the responsibility for Ron's care. Each of these physicians agreed that he needed the surgery but were not, however, willing to schedule it. Apparently they didn't want to be seen as "taking over" his case and making major decisions in the absence of Ron's primary physician. The new physicians also were not very familiar with his medical history and didn't know many important details about his past treatments. Some weren't even aware of the medications he had been taking during the past few weeks. And, in general, they struck Ron as not being very knowledgeable about his disease. He became quite concerned that if he suffered complications they would not be able to manage his care competently.

The delay in scheduling surgery put Ron at risk of developing a hole in his colon. Because of this, he decided that he was no longer getting high-quality care. Luckily he had already done quite a bit of research in the library on his disease. At that time he had located a world-renowned surgeon practicing in a nearby hospital who had helped to develop the type of colon surgery he needed. Ron decided to have an ambulance take him across town so he could be operated on by the well-known surgeon. Because of the danger of serious complications, he made this move quickly, before his first physician even came back to town.

When he arrived at the new hospital Ron quickly had his colon removed, luckily with no problems. He may not have been so fortunate if he hadn't been so knowledgeable and taken a few steps in his own behalf. Remember, he made an effort to learn about the dangers of his condition. He also located one of the best surgeons in the area who had the most experience doing the surgery he needed. Ron did this without any help from his physicians. He also was assertive and self-confident enough to leave the hospital against his physician's wishes in order to receive higher quality care across town.

Some people believe that it's illegal to discharge yourself from the hospital against the wishes of your physician. In Ron's case, his physicians were not at all happy that he decided to take his business somewhere else. But keep in mind that it's a hospital, not a prison. With very few exceptions, people are free to leave whenever they want.

Ron faced a major problem when his primary physician left town during the most critical part of his treatment. His care was put in the hands of less experienced people who were not very familiar with many details of his medical history. They were also somewhat less experienced in treating people with his disease. Unfortunately, it's not at all unusual for people to have to work with new caregivers before treatment is completed. In some cases this is because consumers move to new locations or change to health insurance plans that no longer let them see their original caregivers. Perhaps just as often, one caregiver may leave to fill an assignment in a different part of the hospital or another part of town. Daily changes in schedule may force people to work with different caregivers during different times of the day or week. They could also be moved to another part of the hospital where there are new staff. And, of course, people go away to conferences and on vacation.

Much of the time such changes have a relatively minor impact on consumers' care. In these cases new caregivers are able to provide high quality services quickly without endangering the customer. At other times, it's important to have the same caregivers throughout the entire recovery. As we saw with Ron, this can be important because new practitioners may not know much about your history. Ron's caregivers, in fact, knew very little about his past medical condition. This may have been particularly dangerous in his case because he could have died if one of his new, less experienced physicians made a mistake when he was in such bad physical shape. With Ron then, as with so many people being treated for serious or complicated physical illness, a change in caregivers may mean increased risk and poorer quality care.

Working with one consistent practitioner may also be quite important in other fields. In mental health care, for example, it's often quite destructive for people who develop close relationships with counselors to have to learn suddenly to trust someone else. Nursing home residents may experience a tremendous amount of stress when moved to another facility, or even to another floor of their own building. Some researchers have even claimed that such moves have caused a higher rate of illness and death in those elderly or handicapped people who are forced to relocate.

There may be many times when you will need to insist on more consistency in your care. This could mean staying with the same practitioners and not moving to another location or facility. Because some of these moves are often done simply for the convenience of caregivers, you may have to remind them that such changes are not in your best interests. With a little luck, you will be able to convince them to arrange their schedules so you aren't just jostled from one person to the next. Quite often, for example, nurses' schedules are not set up according to the individual needs of the consumers. Instead, they may be planned according to which nurses happen to be at work that day or how many people are currently being treated in that part of the hospital. You may want to request ahead of time that you receive care from the nurse who has done the most work with you in the past. It's then up to the nursing staff to rearrange their schedules to accommodate your needs. Although sometimes inconvenient for hospital staff, it is quite reasonable for you to make these types of requests if they are likely to result in better care. You could also ask similar courtesies of other practitioners who may need to work with you for the duration of your illness.

If you are not happy with the service, you may be faced with the unpleasant task of trying to make your caregiver comply with your wishes. One researcher (Hayes-Bautista, 1976) has studied the tactics that both consumers and practitioners use when this happens. He reports that people will often first try to argue that the treatment should be changed because it will not help. To accomplish this they may disclose new information. For example, someone might decide to tell a physician that there is a history of cancer in his or her family. The person's motive may be to encourage the physician to conduct a more thorough physical examination or to perform other diagnostic tests. The problem with "deciding" to disclose new information is that everything relating to your problem should automatically be discussed with your caregiver anyway. If you withhold information you may be preventing your practitioner from knowing something that could greatly affect your care. Because of this problem, this strategy is probably most often used by those who have dangerously concealed some information from their caregivers in the first place.

Hayes-Bautista also says that some people make suggestions for treatment, hoping to call caregivers' attention to therapies that may not have been considered. This is likely to be a much safer and productive tactic. It is with this strategy that you might be able to change your care by opening your caregiver's eyes to other, possibly more effective, treatments. After all, you may have spent quite a bit of time in the library learning about the latest research on your illness. Your practitioner, on the other hand, might not have treated anyone with this problem since graduation from school twenty years ago.

An even more tactful approach described by this researcher was to ask a leading question, hoping to direct the professional's thoughts in a more appropriate direction. For example, a person with stomach pains might ask his or her caregiver about the symptoms of a certain disease that she believes she may have. With your own care, this could be an especially good strategy to choose if your caregiver has trouble taking advice. With leading questions, you might be able to have him or her follow your line of reasoning without making it seem like you are directing your own treatment. It's a good way to help many caregivers save face while still insuring that they consider your point of view.

Hayes-Bautista also reports that people sometimes try to change their treatments themselves without the knowledge of their caregivers. Perhaps this is even more dangerous than withholding information. If you do things such as take medication without your practitioner's knowledge or lie about how much you exercise, you are obviously setting yourself up for trouble. This strategy is probably used most often by those who are afraid of confronting caregivers. If you aren't assertive enough to tell your practitioner what you are doing, you may be risking your own neck. Most of the time you would be much better off having a heated argument rather than endangering your health by doing things without your caregivers' knowledge.

When all else fails, some people even threaten to go to different practitioners if their demands are not met (Hayes-Bautista). Although often unpleasant, this may be necessary if you really believe that you can find better service elsewhere. This is always the consumer's option. Unless they are restricted by their insurance plan, they are of course free to bring their business wherever they want.

Hayes-Bautista also described the ways practitioners try to foil consumers who want to make changes in their treatments.

Perhaps the most powerful of these strategies is called the "overwhelming knowledge" argument. Here, the caregiver tries to make the consumer doubt his or her own ability to make decisions about proper treatment. The caregiver may say that he or she studied this problem for years in school and has seen many others with this difficulty. In addition, that practitioner can offer to call in other professionals who will agree with his or her point of view. Notice how this and other tactics are used in the following conversation.

Judy: I would really like you to tell me about the tests I am scheduled to take tomorrow. I don't know what type of tests they are, if they are dangerous, or how they relate to my heart problems. In fact, I'm not convinced that they are necessary.

Mr. Ventricle: (Slightly irritated) I wouldn't worry too much about them if I were you. There is very little risk involved and the discomfort is minimal. If you like, I will ask my colleague Mr. Auricle to visit you if you really feel you need another opinion on this. Besides, there will be technicians with you the whole time to explain what's going on. (Moves toward the door.)

Judy: I really am interested in learning more about the tests now. Exactly what are they and what information do you hope they will provide?

Mr. Ventricle: O.K. but they're very complicated and you really need lots of training to understand. One is called an angiogram and we will use it to look at the blood vessels in your heart. The other is called an EKG and we will use it to see how well your heart beats. We need to do both of these tests or we can't be responsible for what happens to you in this hospital.

Judy: Well, let's start with the angiogram. What will be done to me during that test and what are the risks?

Mr. Ventricle: We will begin by making an incision near your groin into a blood vessel. Then I will insert a long tube in the blood vessel that I will slowly move up towards your heart. When the tube is in place, I'll inject some dye into the arteries in your heart. We can then use an X-ray to look and see if any of the arteries are clogged.

Judy: And what are the risks?

Mr. Ventricle: Very rarely, less than two percent of the time, someone has a serious reaction to the test that could possibly lead to death. You are in fairly good health, though, and we don't have any other reason to expect you will have any problems.

Judy: Is there much radiation involved?

Mr. Ventricle: No.

Judy: Is this test necessary?

Mr. Ventricle: I certainly wouldn't have recommended it if it wasn't.

Judy: You said there was something called an "EGE."

Mr. Ventricle: (Annoyed) No. I said "EKG."

Judy: Oh, that's right. Would you tell me what it is used for and what the risks are?

Mr. Ventricle: We simply want to attach some wires to your chest that will help us keep track of the rate and quality of your heartbeats. If there is a problem that happens when you are in the hospital we will know about it right away. There are no risks.

Judy: O.K. It sounds like these tests would be helpful and the risks are minimal. I guess I'll go through with them. Thanks very much for your time.

Judy had to be very insistent to receive any useful information from this condescending practitioner. His statement "I wouldn't worry too much about them if I were you" quickly gave her the message that he didn't want her to be actively involved in her own care and didn't think she was able to understand her treatment. He also tried to convince her to direct her questions to technicians during the tests. Even the inflections in his voice told her that he didn't want to talk.

Judy did an excellent job of persisting in asking specific questions. These questions eventually made her practitioner give her some useful explanations about the medical tests. She even learned that there was a slight chance of serious complications resulting from the angiogram. At the time that she questioned his advice, she still was willing to learn about his point of view. After all, he was a professional who had much more knowledge and experience than she did.

Along with the overwhelming knowledge argument, Hayes-Bautista points out that caregivers may warn consumers about the possible consequences of not going along with treatments. Recall Mr. Ventricle's rather cryptic warning that he couldn't be responsible for what would happen to Judy if she didn't agree to take both tests. What could be a better strategy than to scare someone to death about what will happen if they don't do as you say? Finally, Hayes-Bautista describes caregivers who act rather chummy with consumers as if they were close acquaintances. Consumers may see this strategy as an attempt to make them go along with the treatment in order to avoid an argument with a "friend."

The strategy of delayed response to requests or questions is another tactic that's often very frustrating to consumers. It's frequently used by caregivers who assist in your treatment but don't have the power to make significant changes in what is done for you. Often these are hospital personnel working under the direction of another caregiver, usually a physician. If you request a change in your care they can't authorize, they should contact your primary practitioner for permission. If they don't really want to change what is being done for you, or if they believe your request is not important, they may try to delay contacting that caregiver until that professional visits you in person. How many of us have heard "The doctor is in with a patient and can't come to the phone" or, "The doctor doesn't seem to be taking any calls right now." This goes on and on while the hospitalized person waits, usually until the next day when that practitioner makes daily rounds.

If your request is a minor one, you should probably just wait it out until your practitioner visits you. If you think your request is more important, you should know that your caregiver can almost certainly be contacted quickly by someone who either: (a) tells the professional's receptionist that there's an urgent problem that needs to be taken care of, or (b) has the credentials to get a phone call through. As for "a," all your nurse or other practitioner has to do is state the importance of speaking with the person in charge. When this is done there is usually a 90% chance of getting through. As for "b," consider the following conversation.

Receptionist: (answering telephone) Hello.

Caller: I would like to speak with Dr. Jones please.

Receptionist: I'm sorry, but Dr. Jones is with a patient right now and can't be disturbed. Can I take a message so he can call you back?

Caller: O.K. Tell him to call me at 123-4567. My name is Dr....

Receptionist: (Interrupting and a bit embarrassed) Oh, I didn't know you were a DOCTOR. Just a minute, I'll put you right through.

Similar conversations happen all the time. The practice of accepting calls from high prestige professionals helps caregivers communicate quickly with each other without being bothered by unnecessary calls. What's important to remember, though, is that by using code words, such as "emergency," your caregiver probably can be contacted very quickly. So, in the event of what you believe to be a serious problem, don't accept repeated excuses that your practitioner can't be reached.

You may notice that you and your caregiver use some of these tactics. If you are satisfied with the results of your talks with that caregiver you will probably stay with your practitioner. If not, the relationship will be so strained you may want to find another professional who will be more willing to listen to and go along with your point of view.

Your practitioner also has the right to suggest that you find another caregiver. Here, the practitioner may be uncomfortable working with you. If this happens your caregiver may find that the poor relationship they have with you prevents you from getting the best care they have to offer. For example, if they don't like you they may find that they tend to schedule fewer appointments with you, return your telephone calls more slowly, or have little time to listen to your descriptions of new symptoms. When this occurs it is their duty to send you to someone else for treatment.

Many practitioners, however, are reluctant to suggest that their customers move on to other caregivers. One reason for this is that they worry it will appear they are abandoning you. They don't want to get a reputation for "dumping" clients without good reason. Because of this problem, the customer is often in the best position to first bring up the possibility of a change in caregivers. When you sense something is wrong in your relationship with your caregiver, discuss it openly with that practitioner. Afterwards, it may still seem that the two of you can't resolve your differences and that those differences affect the quality of your care. In this case you may have to be the first to suggest that you work with someone else. This may help your caregiver avoid worrying about being viewed as someone who abandons clients.

Occasionally consumers are afraid of reprisals from caregivers if they don't get along with their practitioners or if they argue too much. This may be an especially important concern to a seriously ill person who is dependent on others for life-sustaining care. I remember talking with one man who was in the intensive care unit recovering from surgery. Although his care was excellent overall, there was one caregiver who frequently scolded him because he was not recovering as quickly as she had hoped. She called him a "baby" for not walking the day after his operation and for using too much medication to control his pain. She also had a habit of rather roughly bouncing him around in bed when it came time to change his linens. He was concerned that if he complained she would be even less willing to give him as much pain medication as he desired. He was fortunate, though, in that he recovered quickly and was soon transferred out of intensive care, where he no longer saw that professional. Other consumers though, are obviously not so lucky if they are more seriously ill or have to depend on one caregiver for a longer period of time.

Of course, what you decide to do about reprisals will depend on the circumstances of your illness. You may have to rely on an assertive friend or relative to look out for your best interests. If you do decide to confront your caregiver directly, you will probably want to go to great lengths, at least at first, to avoid doing it in front of other people. Some consumers have done this by calling their practitioners into their rooms or by scheduling office visits just to talk about the problem. Public complaints or accusations should always be a last resort.

Sometimes people will suffer at the hands of a caregiver who unintentionally vents frustrations. I remember Sue, a woman who had cancer. As a result of her disease, Sue developed pockets of infection around her lungs that prevented her from breathing normally. She was extremely weak, and didn't have the strength to breathe by herself for any length of time. Consequently, she depended on a respirator to fill her lungs with air. The respirator was connected to her by a tube that was inserted into her neck. Air pumped through this tube went into Sue's lungs and helped her breathe deeply. Without this equipment she would die within a few hours because she would be unable to breathe on her own.

The treatment plan was to "wean" Sue off the respirator gradually as she gained the strength to breathe normally. It was hoped that by the end of the first week she would be able to breathe by herself for an hour each day. Her caregivers planned for this period of time to be gradually increased so that in a few months she wouldn't need the respirator at all. Well, all didn't go as planned. Each time Sue was taken off the respirator for more than an hour she became extremely anxious, feeling as if she would suffocate because of her breathing problems. Each time this happened she insisted that her respirator be started again, much to the disappointment of her caregivers. After two weeks Sue was still using the respirator as much as she had been before. Understandably, her therapists were quite disappointed in her lack of progress. They attributed much of her failure to "nerves." She even was described as a "stubborn patient" who was not willing to "take risks" by learning to breathe on her own. Because of this, one of her caregivers decided that more aggressive measures needed to be taken.

Instead of putting Sue back on the respirator when she requested, her caregiver forced her to breathe by herself for a certain period of time each day. When she tried to ask to be put back on the respirator her caregiver was out of earshot. She was also slower to respond to Sue's requests for other help such as assistance with toileting and moving her pillow. After all "stubborn patients" should, her caregiver reasoned, be encouraged to do as much as possible on their own. Predictably, the result of this new get-tough policy was that Sue became even more upset and anxious when her respirator was turned off. This made her feel more out of control and actually decreased the limited time she spent breathing on her own.

Although the intentions of Sue's caregiver had been good, the new aggressive stance seemed to stem more from the practitioner's frustrations with Sue's lack of progress than on any rational treatment plan. Sue was a constant reminder that her caregivers were unable to help her as they had hoped. In a way, her caregiver was also retaliating against Sue's protest that she was simply too frightened to be taken off the respirator for longer and longer periods of time. In Sue's case, as in many others, she ultimately had to rely on the help of family and friends to intervene. Once they became aware of her situation, they insisted that she be given the right to decide how much time she would spend off the respirator each day. This gave Sue the control again and helped to ease her fears.

With all the problems that do occur, consumers today still often are given exceptionally high quality health care. So, along with your complaints and demands for change, don't forget to express your gratitude for good service. Practitioners usually very much appreciate receiving cards during the holidays or "thank you" notes any time of the year. Although a small box of store-bought chocolates might also be appreciated, stay away from more expensive gifts. Your caregiver may not feel comfortable accepting anything extra from you that's of real value.

Asking Questions

Being able to get helpful answers to questions about health care is a skill that many people lack. Consider the unfortunate man who complained:

"First my ophthalmologist told me what he thought the problem was with my eyesight. It was some sort of nerve disease caused by multiple sclerosis. I'm not sure if he thought it would get worse or not. He also said something about glasses so I think I better buy a pair to see if they help."

This person probably learned little in his meeting with his ophthalmologist. It is clear that he probably did not ask helpful questions or even remember many of the ophthalmologist's replies. Let's look at a few hints that he could have kept in mind when asking about his problem.

1. **Ask specific questions.** Here is how two different people might approach their psychiatric social worker to learn about the probability they will overcome their depression.

   Mr. George: I've been wondering for a long time now about my problem. You see, my depression has lasted a long time and I'm worried that it won't go away even though I'm getting treatment. Tell me, do you think I will ever improve?

   Mr. Caregiver: Well, I know we've been at this for quite a while now and your depression has only gotten a little better. I can't think of anything else that we could do to help. Since you haven't improved very much, I can't predict when you will feel better.

Notice that after asking a general question ("do you think I will ever improve?") Mr. George was given a general reply. In this response, the psychiatric social worker offered no new or useful information. In fact, Mr. George's anxiety may have increased because he could have been left with the impression that his case was a particularly difficult one.

Let's look at how a different consumer may have sought the same information:

Mr. Stevens: I've been concerned lately that my depression may not respond to this treatment. Could you tell me what the chances are that I will eventually recover from depression?

Mr. Caregiver: It's really impossible for me to predict

how you will feel in the future.

Mr. Stevens: Well then, can you tell me what percentage of people receiving this therapy eventually feel better?

Mr. Caregiver: Well, of course everyone responds differently to this therapy and I can't predict exactly how well you will feel in the future. But, I can tell you that the general long-term prognosis for depression is quite good. About 90% of persons with depression feel much better within a year or two even if they get no treatment at all. If they are treated, though, their chances of recovery are better. I would say that about half recover within the first three or four months if they take their medication and also have a chance to discuss ways of changing their behavior.

Mr. Stevens: So from what you have said I understand that there is about a fifty percent chance that I will improve within the next few months.

Mr. Caregiver: That's right, if you respond like most people. But that is something, of course, that I cannot guarantee.

Notice that Mr. Stevens asked specific questions about his chances of feeling better. This forced the practitioner to provide useful and concrete information. As we might expect, many practitioners often are reluctant to "tell the chances" that people will improve. This is usually because it's often so difficult to predict how any individual will do. In this case, though, after some prodding, the psychiatric social worker did tell Mr. Stevens about the number of people who often recover. He qualified his answer though by stating that he couldn't say with any certainty if he would recover from his particular problem.

2. **If you don't understand, ask again.** Everyone has a right to understand their health care. If you are unfamiliar with a word your provider uses or an explanation just doesn't make sense, you have the right to keep asking questions until they are answered to your satisfaction. You aren't a pest if you ask for clarification. Regrettably though, some

practitioners may try to impress you with technical knowledge or language that, unless you have studied about your problem, will leave you quite bewildered. Consider the following conversation:

Technician: In my ten years as an electroencephalograph technician, I have never seen a more conclusive somnographic study. You undoubtedly have bilateral nocturnal myoclonus.

Mr. Fisher: I don't understand what you mean by "somnographic" and "bilateral something or other."

Technician: (With a sigh) Well, "somnographic" basically means a recording taken of your blood pressure, breathing rate, body movements, and so forth while you are asleep. "Bilateral nocturnal myoclonus" is a pattern of nighttime stereotyped leg activity that we record from your anterior tibialis muscle.

Mr. Fisher: What's an "anterior tibialis muscle?"

Technician: A leg muscle.

Mr. Fisher: Then you mean you are concerned that my legs jerk during the night?

Technician: I suppose you could state it that way, yes.

Many people believe they will lose their caregiver's respect if they ask for more explanations to their questions. Actually, the opposite is probably true. Remember that your practitioner may have made a deliberate attempt to confuse you with fancy language. Your practitioner knows that if you do not fully understand your illness you will not be able to make informed decisions about your own health care. As a result, you may make fewer demands and let your caregiver make more of the decisions. In other words, this strategy puts the control in the practitioner's hands. By insisting on full explanations, you regain this control and, in so doing, will likely earn the caregiver's respect.

3. **If possible, prepare your questions in advance.** One of the best ways to insure that you receive the information you need is to spend time preparing your questions well

ahead of time. Many people do this by keeping a list of questions posted on the refrigerator. This way, they are reminded to write down questions as they occur during the day. You could also keep a list in your purse, your briefcase, or anywhere else that is convenient.

4. **Feel free to disagree or present another viewpoint.** Professionals should expect consumers to play an active role in their own health care. When you propose another diagnosis or treatment your practitioner should respect that suggestion. Professionals today are more accustomed to including the customer in this decision making process. In fact, most probably enjoy discussing the pros and cons of other possible diagnoses or treatments.
5. **Study, Study, Study.** Remember how it was purchasing your first car? You may have had almost no idea what to ask the salesperson. In fact, the most technical question you might have come up with may have been to ask if the engine was gasoline or diesel. Only with repeated visits to many showroom floors did you become a more sophisticated shopper. Just as when learning to buy a car, don't expect that you will be able to ask technical or complex health care questions right away. Instead, know that you will be going through a learning process were you will, most likely, stumble along for a while. That's fine. Take your time and learn about your health care by using the library, asking questions, and any other means available.
6. **Practice ahead of time.** It might help you to think through your questions and practice "asking" them even before you meet with your caregiver. You may want to have a friend help you with this practice. Ask your friend to carry on a conversation with you and pretend to be your practitioner. Your friend can tell you if your questions are stated clearly and, when appropriate, make suggestions for improvement.

   Also, if you have a caregiver who discourages you from asking questions, your friend could help you learn to be more assertive. During your practice, your friend, posing as your caregiver, could impatiently look at the clock and use lines like "You need to just trust me and let me make those decisions." It may be especially helpful if your friend knows your practitioner. This way, your friend will know exactly how your caregiver would make it difficult for you during your talk. If your friend isn't familiar with your caregiver, though, you may decide to first reverse roles and demonstrate what you will have to contend with. Then, when your friend knows how your caregiver behaves, you can switch back again and give yourself practice dealing with that behavior.

It is especially important to watch what you do with your body and tone of voice during this practice. Don't speak loudly or do anything else that would make you look angry. Be sure that you look directly at the other person and speak in a firm, self-assured manner. Perhaps your friend will be able to tell you about how you come across and offer suggestions for change.

7. **Don't be a "know-it-all."** Nobody enjoys being talked down to. Instead, most of us like to think that our opinions are respected and that others are lucky to get our advice. Nowhere is this more true than in the health care industry. Your caregiver may have studied about your illness for many years and have a tremendous amount of knowledge. Understandably then, your caregiver may bristle when some "smarty pants" acts as if he or she doesn't know very much. Watch out that you don't say things like "If you lived with this problem for as long as I have you would know..." or "Well I've been doing a lot of reading on this and I think you're wrong when you say...." These statements are almost sure to end any constructive relationship you may have already developed with your practitioner.
8. **Ask when the best time would be to call your caregiver if you have more questions at a later time.**
9. **Ask your questions at the *beginning* of your appointment, not at the end when your caregiver is already half-way out the door.**

In one study (Greenfield, Kaplan, Ware, Yano, & Frank, 1988) people with diabetes were taught to negotiate with their physicians using techniques similar to some of those described above. In fact, the researchers even coached people on how to cope with intimidation by the physician and with their own embarrassment. They found that people who were more active soon had their blood sugar levels under better control than the people who were not as involved in their own care. The authors suggested that the increased sense of control these people experienced may have motivated them to take better care of themselves.

Before starting this study, the authors also guessed that more inquisitive and assertive customers would irritate their physicians. This did not happen. Even though people were more involved in making decisions, this did not seem to hurt the physician-customer relationships.

The most helpful health care professionals will probably tell you just about everything you need to know without you even having to ask. Others, though, will tell you practically nothing unless you persist with your questions. Below are the types of questions that you may need to ask very early on in your treatment when you will be using the library or other sources to learn more about your problem. Your first meetings with your caregiver then are excellent times to ask the questions you need to begin this research.

1. What is the name of my illness?
2. What journals, books, or other publications will tell me more about my problem?
3. Do you have any reading materials that describe this illness?
4. Who are some well known authors who have written about this problem?

After you have this basic information you will probably want to know more details. For example, you may wonder:

1. What percentage of people with my illness get better?
2. When those people do recover, how many are able to

return to work?
3. How many people with this illness lead a normal life again?
4. Is the pain I have now likely to go away?
5. What are the chances that this problem will happen again in the future?
6. What are the dangers of this treatment and how likely is it that they will happen?
7. Is this treatment painful?
8. Are there other therapies I might consider?
9. Exactly how is this treatment likely to help me?
10. Is it possible that I will need more treatment in the future?

Each of these questions may be very important for you to ask in order to fully understand your care. Again, don't be afraid to spend plenty of time talking with your caregiver. It's his or her job to help keep you informed. And, although your caregiver may give you answers, you should always double check them with either another professional or in the library.

One way that caregivers sometimes discourage customers from asking questions could be called "the strategy of the harried and overworked professional." Here, a practitioner will try to look as if he or she is in a terrible rush. This person might dash into the room far behind schedule carrying a stack of charts. When you ask a question, the caregiver may reply briefly and then look at the clock as if late to another appointment. This show is quite intimidating for many who are afraid to take up the busy professional's time. Some are impressed, thinking that it shows his or her services are in demand. I remember hearing about one elderly rural practitioner who usually made his customers wait in his lobby almost an hour. His customers would sit patiently, believing that he was behind schedule because so many others wanted to see him. "He's such a good doctor" they would think, after finishing another issue of National Geographic. Actually he simply arrived to work late every morning, a habit that gave him some extra time to sleep. When he retired, the young man who took his place was almost always on time for his appointments. A few of the townspeople distrusted him though in part because he was never behind schedule and therefore never seemed to be in much demand. As a result, many drove some distance away to another caregiver, who usually made them wait.

Habitual tardiness may mean a number of other things. First, it may indicate that a professional is trying to increase profits by treating more people in less time. Unfortunately, some practitioners overbook themselves and try to see as many people as possible. This sets the stage for mistakes, which are often made when practitioners have too much to do. Also, your practitioner may simply be poor at scheduling, not allowing enough time to treat customers thoughtfully. In either case, it is the customer who may suffer when treated by someone who doesn't spend enough time to do a good job.

The day of a health care professional may also be unpredictable with all sorts of unexpected emergencies. It may be that the caregiver stayed up all night treating someone the night before or was delayed to assist in an emergency. These problems may occasionally put even the most punctual caregiver behind schedule. Such isolated incidents should, of course, just be forgiven. The professionals who consistently appear overworked or are late for appointments are the ones to regard with some suspicion.

For Those Who Have Difficulty Remembering

Some research has shown that almost half of the time people don't take their medications as prescribed. Other people don't exercise properly, eat the right things, or pay attention to important signs of disease. In part, this is caused by problems in understanding or remembering directions. Such difficulties are common and can occur for a number of reasons. First, information about health can often be highly technical and complex. Naturally, it is difficult to understand and retain such details, especially if you are sick or upset. If you are on medication that interferes with memory or concentration you might have some problems. Finally, some people may have long-standing difficulty retaining information. This can lead to embarrassment as well as serious health problems if they can't remember important instructions.

One way to cope with memory problems is to keep written records of what is said during your appointments. Some people in fact, use a form that is filled out during their appointments that contains information about how to care for themselves. This form also may have space for questions to ask the professional. Below is a sample of what your form might look like. Notice that parts of the first section, entitled "My Questions" should be filled out before your appointment. The answers, entered just below each of the questions, are usually written during the appointment. This form is intended only as a guide. Be creative when planning your own form. Perhaps you have health concerns that would make it necessary to add sections on such things as physical exercise, ways to relax, or diet.

Appointment with Dr. Steven Tibia
Date 4/19/91
My Questions:

a. How much can I walk after my knee surgery next week?
(Answer) Plan to stay off my feet as much as possible for a week and wait for instructions from my physical therapist before I start to walk more.

b. Are there any problems after this type of surgery that I should watch for?
(Answer) Watch for any swelling or fever.

c. What medications will I be given in the hospital and are there any common side effects that I might experience?
(Answer) Demerol for pain. No side effects are expected because I have been given that pain killer several times in the past without any complications.

d. What percentage of people having this surgery are able to walk normally again?
(Answer) Almost 100%

e. How many of these surgeries has this surgeon performed and what is the success rate?

(Answer) Over 100 surgeries with all people having good to excellent results.

When to take my medicines:

a. *Pain killers should be taken as needed, up to three tablets a day*

b.

c.

Other instructions:

Plan to take a week off work and walk no more than one block each day until my next appointment.

You can have help filling out this form by your health care professional, or even a friend or relative might attend your appointment to take notes. Another alternative is to ask permission to tape record the appointment. This way you can concentrate fully on the discussion without worrying about writing things down. This might be an especially good solution for those who can't see well or have difficulty writing.

Another frequent problem is not remembering to take medication on schedule. It can be easy to forget to take it on time or become confused about which medication to use. If you are out on the town it can also be a hassle to fumble through your purse or pockets for the correct bottle of pills.

Many people use special medication containers to cope with these difficulties. These are readily available at the pharmacy departments of most drug stores. One type has a built in alarm to help remind you to take your pills. This might be especially helpful if you tend to forget to take your medicine at the correct time of day. Another kind has a series of small compartments, each of which is large enough to hold approximately 20 or 30 average sized pills. At the beginning of the week some people put a day's supply of medication in each compartment. Each section is then labeled with the day of the week its contents are to be consumed. Then, at the end of the day, another compartment will be empty if the correct medicine was taken. Others choose to fill each section with the medicine needed at a particular time of the day. That way, if they need to take their pills four times a day, they might spend a few minutes each morning putting their whole day's medication in four separate compartments. Each compartment is then labeled with the time its contents are to be taken.

Also be sure to ask what your medications look like. Write this information down and keep it with you to avoid making mistakes.

Reading Your Chart

When you are ill, one of your best sources of information is your medical chart, which contains many details about you and your health. If you are hospitalized, it is probably kept outside your room at the nurses' desk. This chart has two main purposes. First, it's a permanent record to help future caregivers know about your illness and treatment. Second, it's a way for all the professionals who treat you to communicate with each other. For example, the physical therapist who sees a hospitalized person in the morning may never even meet that same person's physician who makes rounds in the afternoon. They "talk" to each other about the person through notes that they leave in the chart.

Another reason caregivers make notes in a chart could be to help the hospitalized consumer stay informed. After all, the chart holds valuable information and is an excellent resource for the customer. Unfortunately though, hospital staff often discourage people from reading their charts. One way they do this is to keep the charts far away from the customer's bedside. If a person wants to see their own chart they usually have to wait for a busy nurse to bring it. The caregivers also may not tell consumers that they may read their charts in the first place. Actually, in most states, every hospitalized person is legally entitled to have free access to any information included in their own hospital records. Finally, the hospital personnel may discourage the consumer with the "overwhelming knowledge" argument. Here, they may tell the consumer that they couldn't understand the technical information the chart includes. What they may not add is that the caregivers could easily explain the meaning of the fancy language and confusing numbers.

In fact, when someone does ask to read a chart, nurses or other staff usually first look a bit surprised. Often, after checking with their supervisors they may tell you that it is hospital policy that you need your physician's permission to view these records. Usually they will insist that a nurse or physician be with you at the time. Actually you will probably find it helpful to have someone with appropriate training go through your chart with you. They are often most familiar with the jargon and know how to find the information you need.

If you are just making an office visit, the time that you normally spend reading magazines in the waiting room might be spent more profitably studying your chart. To arrange this, you will probably have to call ahead and make special arrangements with the office staff in the professional's office you are visiting.

Some people even ask to write in their own charts. This is important to them partly because it gives them the chance to express their concerns. It also makes it possible for them to correct mistakes that other people have made and to call caregivers' attention to important topics. It's quite likely though that your caregiver will inform you that the chart is not your property and that you are not allowed to write in it. In this case, you can always ask that an "authorized" person do your writing for you. You may want to sit down with this person and dictate, word for word, what you would like stated in your medical record. Afterwards, read what was written to be certain it is accurate.

But why is it really that important to see your chart? Why not just ask someone how you are doing? One reason is that the people who provide your care may only communicate with each other placing notes in the chart. These notes tend to be sketchy and incomplete. And, about twenty-five percent of them are illegible. Because of this, one caregiver may not know much about what another is doing. Often this will be quite clear to you when you notice that different practitioners make conflicting recommendations for your care. For example, one will be making plans to discontinue your medication at the same time another person is ordering the dosage to be increased.

If these mix-ups occur, you may want to hold a "team

conference." During this meeting all people, including each physician, nurse, and all other therapists meet together with you to discuss your care. You may have friends or family members present if you wish. This conference not only can give you more information about your care, but it may help your practitioners learn how each of the other professionals is treating you. It's possible that when your caregivers first meet in a team conference they will only have vague notions about the services the other practitioners have provided. This may even occur after they have treated you for weeks. In this case it is clear that the caregivers aren't working well with each other and need to coordinate their treatments better.

It's also important for you to read your chart in order to spot mistakes. For example, a caregiver may have prescribed the wrong medication or made an error in reporting your medical history. One recent study (Beers, Munekata, & Storrie, 1990) showed that the medical charts of 60% of hospitalized elderly people contained inaccurate information about their past medications. Other times you may find important information that your caregivers don't know about. I remember one man who told me about his wife's hospitalization for heart problems. She was scheduled to undergo some medical tests and needed an injection of dye to help get a clear X-ray. Unfortunately, the medical staff did not review her chart before the X-ray was taken. Because of this, they did not see that when she had been given this same test years earlier, she had shown a severe allergic reaction to the dye and barely survived. This time she died when the test was given to her again. Her death could have been avoided if the medical staff had read all her records and been aware of the serious side effects of her earlier test.

In one very interesting study (Greenfield, Kaplan, & Ware, 1985) people were encouraged to review their charts. This was done as part of a program designed to teach them to be involved in making decisions about their own care. The researchers found that people were more satisfied with their care if they were more involved in making decisions about their own treatments. Another benefit was that involved people were twice as effective in getting information from their physicians. Also, it was striking that those who reviewed their own charts soon reported fewer physical limitations. This improvement in physical functioning is not that surprising, considering that people who have felt more in control over their treatments have often been shown to do better physically (Greenfield, Kaplan, & Ware, 1985).

Perhaps a good plan is to ask for free access to your chart. When you are first admitted to the hospital, insist that your physician approve this in writing in the "physician's orders" section of your chart. Then nurses and other staff can refer to it at a moment's notice. By doing this you won't have to wait for them to contact your physician each time you want to review your records.

You might also decide that you would like certain friends or relatives to have access to your chart or to be able to get information about your condition from nurses and other caregivers. Again, make your wishes clear when you are first admitted to the hospital. Be certain that your instructions are noted in the chart. You could even allow certain people to call in over the telephone to learn exactly how you are doing. If you do this though, you might want to give special consideration to the information that you don't want released to others. For example, if you have a serious illness you might instruct your caregivers to only discuss your physical comfort and not your chances of survival when they speak with your friends and relatives.

Some caregivers will not understand when you want to review your chart. I remember one professional, when asked to let someone look at her records, brusquely responded "Well O.K. I'll do it because we have nothing to hide." He probably attributed her request to distrust instead of her desire to stay informed. Actually, she wasn't challenging his expertise. Instead, she needed to be able to know enough about her own care to make her own decisions, based upon her own values. And, he certainly wasn't encouraging her to be a good consumer. He also probably felt a bit defensive, knowing that his decisions would be watched. If you encounter this kind of response, don't let it discourage you from reading your chart. Instead, treat this attitude as a relic that still survives from the days when people were encouraged to be less knowledgeable about their health.

There are many times when it is good to have a copy of the information contained in your chart. When you are planning on finding a new caregiver in another city, for example, it could be convenient to have pertinent medical records with you. It might also be wise to always get copies of important documents such as test results, X-rays, or surgical reports just after they first become available to your caregivers. These may be needed years later to see such things as how much a tumor has changed or exactly what was done during your surgery. One problem in relying on a hospital or clinic to provide them at that later date is that some facilities throw records away after just a few years. Other times they get lost. If either these things were to happen you probably would be out of luck if you hadn't requested copies of them earlier.

CHAPTER 5

Consumer Rights and Problems

"Trust in god but tie up your camels."
—Unknown

Consumer Rights

When you are hospitalized you have certain rights. Many states have, in fact, written "Bills of Rights" that specify the type of treatment to which all hospitalized people are legally entitled. If your state has adopted such a bill, you will probably be able to get a copy of it from your hospital or caregiver. One of these bills was adopted by the State of Minnesota to insure that every hospitalized person's "civil and religious liberties, including the right to independent personal decisions and knowledge of available choices, shall not be infringed...." Although this particular bill has not been formally adopted by all states, it is clearly pertinent to all people being treated in the hospital. Below is a list of each of the specific rights contained in the bill that relate to hospitalized persons as well as an (often shortened) explanation of each of those rights. Many of these rights have already been discussed at some length earlier in this book. Others will be discussed later in this chapter.

Patient's Bill Of Rights

1. Information About Rights. Patients shall, at admission, be told that there are legal rights for their protection during their stay at the facility or throughout their course of treatment....
2. Courteous Treatment. Patients have the right to be treated with courtesy and respect for their individuality....
3. Appropriate Health Care. Patients have right to appropriate medical and personal care based on individual needs.
4. Physician's Identity. Patients [or their guardians] shall have or be given, in writing, the name...of the physician

responsible for coordination of their care....

5. Relationship With Other Health Services. Patients who receive services from an outside provider are entitled...to be told the identity of the provider....
6. Information About Treatment. Patients shall be given by their physicians complete and current information concerning their diagnosis, treatment, alternatives, risks, and prognosis as required by the physician's legal duty to disclose. This information shall be in terms and language the patients can reasonably be expected to understand. Patients may be accompanied by a family member or other chosen representative. This information shall include the likely medical or major psychological results of the treatment and its alternatives....
7. Participation in Planning Treatment. Notification of Family Members:
   a. Patients shall have the right to participate in the planning of their health care. This right includes the opportunity to discuss treatment and alternatives with individual caregivers, the opportunity to request and participate in formal care conferences, and the right to include a family member or chosen representative....
   b. If a patient who enters a facility is unconscious or comatose or is unable to communicate, the facility shall make reasonable efforts...to notify either a family member or a person designated in writing by the patient as the person to contact in an emergency that the patient has been admitted to the facility. The facility shall allow the family member to participate in treatment planning....
8. Continuity of Care. Patients shall have the right to be cared for with reasonable regularity and continuity of staff....
9. Right to Refuse Care. Competent patients shall have the right to refuse treatment....
10. Experimental Research. Written, informed consent must be obtained prior to patient's participation in experimental research. Patients have the right to refuse participation....

11. Freedom From Abuse. Patients shall be free from mental and physical abuse...Every patient shall also be free from non therapeutic chemical and physical restraints....
12. Treatment Privacy. Patients shall have the right to respect and privacy as it relates to their medical and personal care program. Case discussion, consultation, examination, and treatment are confidential and shall be conducted discreetly. Privacy shall be respected during toileting, bathing, and other activities of personal hygiene....
13. Confidentiality of Records. Patients shall be assured confidential treatment of their personal and medical records, and may approve or refuse the release to any individual outside the facility....
14. Disclosure of Services Available. Patients shall be informed...of services which are included in the facility's basic per diem or daily room rate and that other services are available at additional charges....
15. Responsive Service. Patients have the right to a prompt and reasonable response to their questions and requests.
16. Personal Privacy. Patients shall have the right to every consideration of their privacy, individuality, and cultural identity as related to their social, religious, and psychological well-being.
17. Grievances. Patients may voice grievances and recommend changes in policies and services to facility staff and others of their choice....
18. Communication Privacy. Patients may associate and communicate privately with persons of their choice and enter and...leave the facility as they choose...
19. Personal Property. Patients may retain and use their personal clothing and possessions as space permits, unless to do so would infringe upon rights of other patients, and unless [dangerous] for documented medical, safety, or programmatic reasons....
20. Services for the Facility. Patients shall not perform labor or services for the facility unless those activities are included for therapeutic purposes and appropriately goal-

related in their individual medical record.

21. Protection & Advocacy Services. Patients shall have the right of reasonable access...to any available rights protection services....

Try to remember these basic rights as you continue reading this book. As you become comfortable with them, you will probably be able to see how they could apply to many people, both in and out of the hospital.

Research

During the course of your treatment you may be asked to participate in one or more research projects. These studies are done to learn more about certain treatments or illnesses. Such studies are essential to the advance of scientific understanding of health problems. Because of the importance of research, it's everyone's duty to consider helping any investigator who asks them to participate in one of these projects.

If you are asked to take part in a study, there are a few questions you should ask before you agree to help. First, and perhaps most importantly, you should know whether you will face any risks as a result of your participation in the research. This is because some studies might expose you to a dangerous drug or procedure. Others may ask you questions or do things that you may find embarrassing or consider to be an invasion of your privacy. Still other projects involve withholding treatment that could prove beneficial. On the other hand, there are often benefits to participating in a research project. It may give you the chance to receive a treatment not normally available to the public. It will be up to you to weigh the pros and cons and decide for yourself whether the risks or discomforts (if any) of taking part in the study are worth the benefits you or others may receive.

Ron, the man described earlier who had his colon removed, had to make such a decision. A few weeks after his surgery he went in for an exam to determine whether or not a new "colon" that the surgeon had constructed out of intestine was working correctly. The basic idea of the test was to first have air pumped into his rectum through a tube. The hospital's fancy new X-ray equipment would then be used to determine whether or not his new plumbing was the correct size and in the proper place. The day that he had the test, however, a large group of female professionals interested in the X-ray equipment paid a surprise visit to the hospital. After he already had his pants down, one of them asked if they all could be allowed to observe his examination. They were intending to do research on the suitability of that X-ray equipment for their own customers.

Ron told them "no." He decided that he would be too embarrassed and uncomfortable displaying his bare behind to all those women. To him, this embarrassment wasn't worth the possible benefits of helping visitors learn more about the X-ray equipment.

If you decide to cooperate with any researcher, you should be given a "Research Consent Form" to sign before you begin the project. This form should describe the study in detail and also tell you about the foreseeable risks and benefits. If your name is to be kept confidential (not published along with the research data) this should also be explained. The consent form should contain the telephone number of a person you can contact in the event of a research-related injury or if you have other questions about the project. Furthermore, it should tell you that you can drop out of the project at any time with no penalty.

How To Spot a Quack

"Pay no attention to the man behind the curtain."
*—Wizard (*The Wizard of OZ, *1939)*

Billions of dollars are spent each year on treatments that don't work or are dangerous. People fall for these "cures" for many reasons, including low educational level, slick marketing strategies, and their own desperate searches for help. To avoid being conned into a treatment that could harm you both physically and financially, you should know about some of the things that might tip you off that your practitioner is a crook. Below is a selection of some of the things that should concern today's consumer who lives by the principle of "buyer beware."

1. **Products that are illegal in one or more states.** Quite often treatment may be considered dangerous or ineffective by authorities in one area of the country. Officials in that area may outlaw the practice, forcing some quacks to move their offices. Beware if you must travel to another state to be treated. Most likely the caregivers you would work with will explain that their treatment is illegal in some areas because it isn't yet "appreciated" or "understood" by professionals in other parts of the country.
2. **Products for which insurance companies will not pay.** Although insurance companies can be unreasonable and refuse to pay for care that is necessary and effective, they nevertheless are aware of most legitimate forms of treatment. If they balk at the treatment you desire, at least give some thought to the fact it just might not be a therapy that has been shown safe and effective by scientific studies.
3. **Before-after pictures.** These are usually one of the cheapest forms of deceptive advertising. They often use touched up pictures that don't show the true results of their treatment. Even if the pictures are genuine, they may just show the improvement that occurs in a small minority of people using their product or services. Companies that sell diet pills, which are probably totally ineffective for long term weight loss, are notorious for using these ads.
4. **Claims that they have skills not possessed by any other caregiver.** If your practitioner says that he or she alone has the ability to cure your ills, that professional is almost certainly a liar. Reputable caregivers with the same specialty area share a common body of knowledge and it is almost never the case that only one practitioner could effectively treat your problem. Perhaps the only exception to this would be in the case of a new experimental treatment that is just being developed and used on a few people. In this case though, you should be given forms (described earlier) to sign explaining the nature of the research project.
5. **Attempts to get you to solicit business for them.** Some

practitioners actually have posted the names of their customers in their waiting rooms if those customers have sent family or friends to them for treatment. Other unscrupulous caregivers may offer you a discount on your care if you bring them business.

6. **Inappropriate physical or sexual contact.** It is never acceptable for a caregiver to have sexual contact with a customer. Sometimes a practitioner will even try to convince someone that sex is an accepted and necessary part of treatment. If this occurs, the consumer should immediately report that caregiver to any professional guild to which that caregiver may belong. In some states such sexual contact is illegal (Schoener, et al, 1989) and should be reported to the police. It is quite possible that that practitioner is victimizing others as well. These sexual relationships may be particularly destructive to consumers of mental health care who, because they may going through emotionally difficult times, can be particularly vulnerable to the advances of a therapist.
7. **Claims that a medicine or service will cure many types of problems.** If someone offers you a product that they claim will cure everything from hemorrhoids to gallstones, use your common sense and stay away.
8. **Claims that a medicine or service will cure a problem that doesn't seem related to the treatment.** One practitioner's sign stated that "spinal adjustments" would help ward off colds and flu. Over the telephone she said that spinal manipulation probably affected peoples' immune systems. Further, it was her impression that this treatment had resulted in a reduction in colds and flu in her previous clients. She went on to explain that there was no scientific evidence supporting her claim, a fact she said she discussed with each person before she offered treatment.
9. **Criticisms of other caregivers.** Sometimes unethical practitioners boast about their ability to cure illnesses that other caregivers are unable to treat. In the process, they

may also make attacks on other professional guilds. When caregivers do this not only can it be unprofessional, but it often is done to disguise their own inadequacies.

What To Tell Employers

Discrimination by employers is one of the great injustices sometimes encountered by people who have already struggled with illness. This may occur if your employer believes that you have an illness that has the potential to interfere with your job performance. Perhaps one example of this is the survivor of cancer, whose supervisor is concerned that any recurrence of the disease might keep her away from her desk. During this time her office would be empty and a co-worker would have to do her job. It might be easy for the employer to simply find someone else for the job and avoid this risk.

Another example is the person who has been treated for mental illness. In some cases the employer again risks keeping an employee who may be nonproductive for long periods of time. Sometimes this might be an even more difficult situation because supervisors, like many people, can look at mental illness somewhat differently than "regular" health problems. This stigma, which is often attached to certain emotional problems can further encourage discrimination.

These problems may leave the employee in a bind when deciding what information to give an employer. On the one hand, the employee might risk encountering problems on the job by being totally honest. If, however, the employee decides to withhold some of the details or lie about the illness, the employee might be fired for dishonesty.

Your decision should depend upon a number of things. First, is your illness really likely to interfere with your job? If it isn't, can you find a caregiver to emphasize this in a letter to your employer? You may also need to think about how your employer has responded to other employees who have faced similar difficulties in the past. Ask others in your work place how the boss treated them if they have been sick. If you are concerned, see an attorney. There are laws that protect you from discriminatory firing.

Also, when you talk with your employer you may be concerned about confidentiality regarding your illness. There are many circumstances where you won't want your coworkers to know the grisly details of your health problems. If so, be sure to discuss this with your employer and insist that your privacy be respected. You may also have a legal right to confidentiality so again the services of an attorney might be helpful.

Living Wills

Most states have passed laws that help people have some control over their own medical treatments if they ever are unable to make decisions for themselves. In this legislation, states have responded to the wishes of citizens who wanted to have more to say about their lives and also to spare others the job of making agonizing ethical decisions in their behalf. This control has been given to consumers in the form of living wills. In these wills, people decide such things as what heroic measures, if any, should be taken to prolong their lives if they are terminally ill. For example, the comatose victim of an automobile accident who has no chance of regaining consciousness may request that caregivers keep him or her alive at all costs, no matter how many machines or dollars it takes to keep the heart pumping. Others instruct caregivers to discontinue treatment in similar circumstances.

This legislation also benefits caregivers. The living wills may give them clear guidelines on how to care for people who are no longer able to make their own decisions. These guidelines protect them from liability in the event that their treatment decisions are questioned at a later time.

A belief in peoples right-to-die apparently has been growing in the U.S.A Louis Harris Poll found that 85% thought terminally ill people should be able to tell their caregivers to let them die rather than prolong their lives (see Mehling, 1985). Contrast this to the general attitude among physicians twenty years ago, when any suggestion that life shouldn't be extended was usually seen as an inexcusable violation of the Hippocratic Oath.

Living wills create the opportunity to make your wishes known on many topics other than just whether or not to prolong your life. With them, you could choose a person to make decisions in your behalf. This is usually a friend or relative who understands your feelings and would help direct your treatment in the event that a situation nobody anticipated occurs. For example, one of your priorities might be for your body organs to be made available for transplantation at the time of your death. The person then might insist your organs be transplanted soon after your death and long before they have had a chance to deteriorate. Other things that could be included in a living will are directions on how much pain medication to use, which caregivers you want to employ, or the experimental treatments to which you would be willing to submit.

It's probably very important for you to spend enough time explaining your wishes to the person you choose to direct your care. Tell them in detail what should be done for you in the event of many different situations. Be sure that they have a good "feel" for your preferences and reasoning. Once they understand your reasoning they should be able to apply those same general principles to many different kinds of decisions that may be made in the future. In fact, one good way to do this might be to invite your family, friends, or clergy to participate in the writing of your will.

It should be clear that making a living will not only takes a great deal of soul searching but also much knowledge about the treatments that would be available to you in the future. This is another reason to be a well-informed consumer. The person who knows about the many different treatment options is usually going to be better able to choose the care that is most consistent with his or her own wishes.

If you are interested in making a living will it would probably be best to do the whole thing with the help of an experienced attorney. If that's too expensive you could obtain a preprinted form for a living will from the Concern for Dying/Society for the Right to Die. Their address is 250 West 57th St., New York, N.Y. 10107. The form they send you should be drafted to take into consideration the specific laws concerning living wills in your state. If you do use one of the preprinted forms, it still might be a good idea to hire an attorney to read through the finished product. Keep in mind, these wills are not written in stone. They may be altered or revoked at any time should your wishes change. Be sure to give a copy to your caregiver to include in your medical record as well as one to any friends, relatives, or clergy who might help carry out its instructions. Don't keep your only copy locked away in your safe deposit box because others may not have access to it if you are incapacitated.

Your Hospital Bill

If you think it was difficult to understand articles written about your illness, just wait until you try to decipher your hospital bill. This will probably be sent to you shortly after your discharge. You will want to be sure to ask for an itemized copy of your bill, especially if you are responsible for paying part of it yourself. It is likely that it will be anywhere from five to fifteen pages long and full of unfamiliar names of medications, tests, and other services the hospital provided. You will probably have to ask for help from a health care practitioner to understand it all. Don't be surprised if it shows that you have been charged $2.50 for each aspirin tablet or $4 for a small piece of gauze. After all, the hospital may remind you that there are a lot of overhead costs to pay for. But do look out for other obvious mistakes. Some people (Findlay, 1990) recommend that you keep a record of the services that were provided to you during your stay. For example, you may want to keep track of the number of hours you spent in the operating room (at $500 an hour) or of the amount of time that your psychiatrist actually spent with you in your room (at $125 an hour). Simple mistakes can quickly add up at these prices. Also watch for charges for medications that you cannot remember.

If there is a problem, first contact the hospital's business office. In most cases they will be able to explain things to your satisfaction or correct any problems. If that doesn't work you might ask your insurance company to review the charges. They may be especially interested in catching mistakes because they probably will be responsible for paying a large chunk of the costs. You might also try complaining to your caregivers or directly to the hospital administration. An attorney might be contacted as a last resort. (Findlay, 1990).

Part 2

Looking Inside, a Change in Perspective

The first part of this book emphasized understanding and changing things that happen around you. In it, you were helped to deal with others to increase your chances of getting the best care. In this second section, I will focus on you. As in earlier chapters, it is written to help you have better treatment, but now the primary caregiver is yourself. You are the only person who can know your own thoughts and feelings. In this sense, you are the best expert on helping yourself. Do not miss the opportunity to use your expertise. If you do, you may neglect some of the most powerful and important parts of your treatment.

Please remember that many of the problems described in this book can be life threatening. Be sure to seek medical care from a competent professional if you believe you may have a medical problem. This book was not designed to be a self-treatment manual or as a medical guide.

CHAPTER 6

Keeping Comfortable

God will not drive flies away from a tailless cow.
–African proverb

Controlling Pain, Anxiety, And Other Problems

Even with the sophisticated medical technology available today, sick people still often endure many uncomfortable physical symptoms. For those who are recovering from surgery, undergoing a medical test, or even having an injection, the discomfort may only last a short while. Others, though, have to suffer much longer. Perhaps they have back pain that cannot be cured with surgery. Or, they may have pain caused by tumors or many other illnesses.

In some cases physical discomfort can actually interfere with medical treatment. One person was being treated with medication to cure her cancer. She received monthly injections of a powerful cancer fighting drug designed to attack her cancerous tumors. Unfortunately, this medication also caused her to feel nauseated for days. The medications that were prescribed to control these symptoms were not very effective, and made her so groggy that she slept most of the time she was in the hospital. In fact, she was so sleepy that she usually needed to spend an extra day in the hospital until the effects of her medication wore off. After six months of this therapy, she finally decided she could no longer endure the treatment. She asked to have her cancer-fighting medication changed to something that would not cause such severe uncomfortable side effects. Unfortunately, if her caregivers had changed her medications there would have been less of a chance of curing her disease.

Instead of giving her different medication, her practitioners recommended that she try to learn to control the side effects of her cancer-fighting medicine without drugs. After some thought, she took their advice and learned to relax her body and distract herself. With some practice she soon felt so much better that she no longer needed large doses of medication to help her feel comfortable. Because she didn't take so many drugs, she was more alert and was able to leave the hospital sooner after her treatments.

These techniques also gave her choices in ways to control her discomfort. These choices were very important to her. They helped her gain more control over what was done to her body. She didn't have to passively accept every pill and injection that was offered to her, but instead could help herself feel better using methods that she chose. This was an especially welcome change for her since her cancer had already made her feel so vulnerable and out of control.

Whatever the cause of your discomfort, it may be helpful to have the input of caregivers with a variety of areas of expertise. Some will suggest medical treatments such as medication or surgery, while others will instruct you in the use of a range of self-management techniques for control of pain and anxiety. These are usually not medical treatments but instead are ways that people change their thoughts or behaviors to reduce their pain. Many people who have used these self-management approaches have been able to rely less on medication for pain or anxiety control. There have also been a number of studies (Devine & Cook, 1986) showing that some people using these strategies have felt better sooner and were able to spend less time in the hospital.

Self-management pain control techniques are the only safe and effective methods of pain relief for some people. Most often, this is because people who have chronic pain that lasts months or years find that they eventually develop a tolerance to their pain control medications. After a while they need to take more and more of them to get the same relief. Soon, they are addicted and experience negative side effects due to the high doses of medication. Clearly, they need to find another way to reduce their pain.

The self-management techniques you choose should be selected with careful thought about your personality style. What works well for one person may be a flop for the next. There are two broad categories of personality style to consider. First, some people think logically and scientifically. They prefer to see order in the world around and have difficulty tolerating things that don't seem to follow their organized system of rules. In contrast, others like to let their minds wander to whatever happens to catch their interest at the moment.

The first group, let's call them the "scientists," go from one organized and "logical" thought to the next. In this sense they are just like Mr. Spock on Star Trek. This is much different from the style of others, who find themselves lost in vivid and colorful daydreams. While the scientists may "think like a typewriter" (verbally) the others may "think like a T.V." (visually). Predictably, members of each of these groups may choose vastly different strategies to control discomfort. While the scientists may prefer more regimented techniques like diaphragmatic breathing, people who think more visually usually prefer to take advantage of their already vivid imaginations by using imagery (both techniques are described below).

A few people feel anxious when they let their minds "wander." For these people, techniques that encourage them to let themselves think about whatever comes to mind can cause distress. Often this is because when their thoughts do wander, they think about some frightening event. These people can be described as having a high desire for control. They try to control their thoughts and prevent themselves from thinking about whatever it is that raises their anxiety. People like this should not try to use techniques that may increase their anxiety. Instead, they should use other, more structured, techniques that will work better for them.

Others avoid relaxation techniques that make them pay attention to parts of their bodies that are uncomfortable. For example, the breathing exercises described later in this chapter might encourage a person with a stomach ulcer to concentrate more on the abdomen. This could cause even more pain than was felt before learning the relaxation technique.

When reading through the pain and anxiety control techniques listed below, try to remember what has worked (or not worked) for you in the past. Perhaps you have developed skills in meditation, a discipline that many find to be very calming. You may want to give special consideration to those strategies that are similar to the meditation that helped you in the past. If your meditation was a disaster though, you might want to consider trying something radically different that may have a better chance of helping you. Also, keep in mind that different techniques may work better at different times in your life. So experiment with a variety of methods to find those that will help you the most right now.

If you do try some new techniques, remember that at first they may feel strange and uncomfortable. They might make you aware of body sensations that you have not noticed before, or take a lot of time and concentration. If so, you may need to practice them for a while before they feel natural and actually help you with your problems.

Occasionally people have physical problems that make it difficult or dangerous for them to learn some of the relaxation exercises described below. For example, those with back injuries might notice an increase in pain when they practice techniques that require them to tighten and relax their back muscles. Others may have problems breathing that prevent them from learning breathing skills safely. If you suspect that you may have a physical problem that would make it dangerous for you to do any of these exercises, be careful. Before you begin talk with a health care professional who could warn you about any risks.

This chapter was written to provide you with a smorgasbord of techniques to control pain and anxiety. Pick and choose those that fit you the best. If needed, make changes in the strategies so they are better tailored to your needs. If you want help learning to use them, seek a health care professional trained in these methods. These techniques are most commonly taught by psychologists, although people with specialties in nursing, dance/movement therapy, social work, and other fields may be skilled instructors. Many of these specialists are available in even the smallest hospitals or in communities with just a few thousand residents.

When you practice these relaxation exercises remember to keep outside distractions to a minimum. Unplug the telephone, send the kids out to play, and lock the door. It often helps to wear comfortable clothing that doesn't bind. Also, many people find it helps to keep their arms and legs uncrossed. After practicing relaxation techniques, don't immediately sit upright. If you are lying down, roll on your side and use your arms to get up slowly.

And finally, remember that sometimes these techniques don't work. You may find that medication is the best way to control your symptoms. If this is the case, don't criticize yourself for having "failed." Instead, it will be more helpful for you to practice these strategies with a spirit of permissiveness. Don't expect yourself to be an expert at them right away. If any of these techniques work at all, they may take several weeks before you notice any real improvement in your comfort. For this reason, you may want to practice them well ahead of time if you think you will need them in the future. Many people find that first practicing them a month or so before they are needed gives them enough time to learn the strategies that work best for them.

Specific Techniques

1. **Diaphragmatic breathing.**

   Especially suited for those who:

   a. Think more verbally than visually.
   b. Have a higher need for control.
   c. Have problems with muscle tension that may cause headache or back pain.
   d. Have trouble with anxiety.
   e. Have learned similar breathing techniques while in sports, playing a musical instrument or singing.

Diaphragmatic breathing is a technique commonly used to help people relax many different groups of muscles. Perhaps it is most often practiced to loosen the shoulders, chest, and upper back. This is because people who have pain such as backache or headache frequently feel much better when the painful areas are relaxed. This probably happens because excess muscle tension often increases pain. By getting rid of that tension, the pain is reduced or eliminated. Diaphragmatic breathing is one of the relaxation techniques that works the fastest, with people often noticing improvement within a few minutes of learning to breathe correctly.

The diaphragm is a sheet of muscle that separates the thorax (which holds the heart, lungs, and other organs) from the abdomen (which contains the stomach, intestines, etc.). It is attached to the ribs in front and on the sides. In back, it is attached to the spinal column. The diaphragm helps you inhale by pulling downward and decreasing air pressure in the lungs. This draws air into the lungs. Also, as the diaphragm moves down it tends to gently pull the shoulders down with it. You can feel this for yourself when you practice your diaphragmatic breathing. You will notice that as you breathe using the diaphragmatic techniques described below, your shoulders tend to drop. This often quickly relaxes the muscles in the shoulders, chest, and upper back.

We also breathe by expanding our chests. In this case, muscles on the ribs move the chest out in front and on the sides. Again, this lowers the pressure in the lungs and draws in air. Many people believe that when we breathe primarily by expanding our chests (as opposed to by using our diaphragms), the muscles in the shoulders and neck tighten. You might notice this when you are under stress. It's at these times that you are likely to expand your chest more as you breathe. As your chest expands it lifts the shoulders up and causes the muscles along the tops of the shoulders to tighten.

The point of diaphragmatic breathing therefore, is to learn to breathe primarily by using your diaphragm, rather than by expanding your chest. This should help the muscles in the shoulders, chest, and upper back loosen, and could be a major step in helping you to feel more relaxed.

To begin, sit in a comfortable chair. Reclining in a bed or on a couch may also work but could change your chest movements and make it a bit more difficult to learn this technique. Once you are settled, put one hand on your navel and the other higher on your chest, right in the middle of your rib cage. Then spend about five minutes observing and listening to your breathing pattern. Don't try to change your breathing yet. The first goal of this exercise is to find out what parts of your chest and abdomen move the most when you breathe. Pay attention to which hand moves the most as you inhale and exhale. Most people find that the hand resting on their chest moves more than the lower hand. They are breathing "up high" and, in so doing, are taking shallow breaths. Many of these people notice that when their upper chest is the main part moving with each breath their shoulders follow. The result is that with each breath the shoulders and upper back tighten. This may cause an increase in shoulder and back tension leading to headache, backache, and a sore, stiff feeling. After you have observed your "normal" breathing, try to breathe more deeply, this time using your diaphragm. Stick out your belly with each breath you take in. When you do this you will notice that your lower hand, resting on your navel, will move more than your top hand. Your second goal should be to keep your top hand almost perfectly still. When this happens, you will notice that your shoulder and upper back muscles quickly become more relaxed. Those of you who learned to play musical instruments or participated in choir would probably recognize this type of breathing. Your conductor may have taught you to breathe using your "stomach" to improve your breath support. Others who have participated in sports or learned techniques such as yoga may have had similar experiences. After a while you will get the feel of breathing like this and no longer need to keep you hands on your stomach and chest. Also, be sure not to breathe too quickly or you will feel lightheaded.

Although you may notice rapid improvement in your muscle tension, pain, and even anxiety, the changes will probably be short lived. Just five or ten minutes after you stop practicing you discomfort could return. The problem then, is that when you stop breathing "diaphragmatically" your muscles tighten. The only way to stay relaxed all the time then is to breathe deeply, using your diaphragm, all the time. To do this, you should begin by practicing your breathing exercises at least twenty times each day. Each practice session should last a minute or two. Although this might seem like a lot of work, keep in mind that you can and, in fact should, continue your normal daily activities while you are practicing. You might practice while you are talking on the telephone, driving your car, enjoying a movie, or arguing with your children. It's important that you practice throughout the day to train yourself to breathe diaphragmatically all the time. If you wait until you are under a lot of stress to practice your breathing it's probably too late. Your muscles are already tight and uncomfortable and it may be difficult to relax. If, however, you have already been breathing correctly it is less likely that you will ever develop these problems in the first place.

When you first practice breathing, you may find that you need help remembering to do it throughout the day. Some people who have watches with alarms set them to go off every twenty minutes or so. The alarm is a signal to practice breathing. One advantage of using a watch alarm is that it will sound while you are doing a wide variety of activities. This should train you to use your breathing skills all day long. If you don't have a watch alarm or are concerned that it would be distracting, try placing reminders around your home and work place. Many people do this by purchasing small brightly colored stickers to place in locations they are likely to see throughout the day. For example, the refrigerator door, the edge of a rear view mirror in a car, or a watchband are good places to put them.

2. **Progressive muscle relaxation.**
   Especially suited for those who:
   a. Think more verbally than visually.
   b. Have a higher need for control.
   c. Have muscle tension that contributes to headache or chronic back pain.

Progressive muscle relaxation, first described in 1929 (Jacobson, 1929), is another "tried and true" relaxation technique. It's well researched and has been shown to be one of the most effective ways to help people reduce their own anxiety, pain, and muscle tension. There are two main goals when practicing this technique. First, it is designed to help you recognize when your muscles are tight. This is vitally important for many people who have endured muscle tightness and tension for years. After so long a period, they often don't notice muscle tension. Instead, they believe that it's normal for shoulders to feel uncomfortable. For them, the first step is to realize that their high level of muscle tension is hurting them and should be changed. In fact, once they have learned to recognize the tension they can be taught to use it as a signal that they are under too much stress. While the first goal then is to recognize that tension exists, the second is to do something about it by relaxing the muscles.

Begin your practice by lying on your back on a chair, couch, or bed. Close your eyes and pay attention to your body. After a few minutes concentrate on the sensations in your feet. You may feel some muscle tightness or relaxation in the feet. There may be a cool draft blowing over the feet and warmth below them where they rest on the bed or are inside of your shoes. Whatever the sensations are, pay close attention to them. Next, tighten the muscles in the feet for about ten seconds. Be careful not to tighten them for too long if you have a tendency to develop muscle cramps. Then, say the word "relax" to yourself. As you do so, let your feet relax for another twenty seconds. Again be aware of the feelings coming from the feet. The important thing is that you recognize in what ways the feet feel different when they are tightened than when they are relaxed. Learn to be aware of the different sensations coming from your body when it is in various states of relaxation. Repeat this process once more, saying the word "relax" to yourself just before letting your feet loosen.

When you have tightened and relaxed the muscles in the feet twice, move your attention higher. Now concentrate on the calves. Again, begin by paying close attention to all of the sensations coming from the calves. Have a good idea how tight or relaxed they feel. As you did with your feet, now tighten the calves, using the word "relax" as your cue. After ten seconds, relax those muscles for twenty more seconds. Then tighten them again and let them relax just as you did the first time.

Proceed in this same manner, tightening and relaxing all the muscles in your body, focusing on one muscle group after another. These groups might be a) the upper legs, buttocks, and thighs, b) the lower abdomen, c) the upper chest and shoulders, d) the arms and hands, and e) the head, neck, and face. If you notice that you have more muscle tension in one particular part of the body you may want to tighten and relax those muscles more than twice.

You should practice this exercise once or twice each day, for about fifteen minutes at a time. Again, try to do it at more or less random times during the day when you are able to take a break from your other activities. Don't put it off until just before bedtime or always do it over the noon hour. Practicing it at many different times will make it easier for you to learn to relax throughout the day. After a few weeks you should be able to say the word "relax" to yourself and notice that it quickly helps reduce your muscle tension as well as your pain and anxiety.

3. Sensory awareness. Especially suited for those who:

a. Have problems with anxiety.
b. Have difficulty "turning off" their thoughts when they are doing other relaxation exercises.

Occasionally, people report that they can't "stop thinking" when they are practicing relaxation. Some caregivers have found that these people need a form of relaxation that captures their attention. Goldfried and Davison (1976) described such a technique that they called "relaxation by sensory awareness." It requires people to frequently shift their attention and concentration. It often helps people relax quickly, especially if they can become "lost" in thought when they practice this exercise. Goldfried and Davison noted that the script for this exercise can easily be recorded and played to the person who is learning relaxation. Below is a sample script, which gives suggestions for this exercise.

Sit back or lie down in a comfortable chair, on a bed, or on a couch. If you have eyeglasses you may want to remove them. You may also want to take off your shoes, loosen your belt, or your collar. Close your eyes now and let your body sink down and become more and more comfortably relaxed and at ease. But as you do this, be sure to pay attention to my words. Concentrate intently on everything I say, not letting anything escape your notice. Pay attention to every inflection in my voice. Notice each time the pitch rises, lowers, or stays the same. Be aware of when I talk more slowly or more quickly. Let nothing go unnoticed. But pay even closer attention to those things I tell you to think about. When I ask you a question, give it your full attention. Use all of your powers of concentra-

tion to think about the answer. You don't need to give an answer though. Just think about the question and give the answer to yourself.

- Are you aware of the heaviness that is coming over your entire body? (Wait five seconds)
- Have you noticed how your breathing is slowing down? (Wait five seconds)
- Can you concentrate enough to notice that there is a very slight twitch in at least one finger? (Wait five seconds)
- Can you imagine the distance between your chin and your feet? (Wait five seconds)
- Is it possible for you to be aware of exactly how far your stomach moves each time you breathe? (Wait five seconds)
- Can you feel the muscles in your lower back loosen with each breath? (Wait five seconds)
- Is it possible for you to imagine what it would look like to gaze at a brightly colored balloon? (Wait five seconds)
- Can you visualize the distance between your shoulder blades? (Wait five seconds)
- Is it possible to tell which is moving the most when you breathe, your stomach or your chest? (Wait five seconds)
- Can you imagine yourself floating comfortably in a warm pool of water? (Wait five seconds)
- Can you imagine the shape of your hands? (Wait five seconds)
- Can you imagine a beautiful sunset with colors of purple, red, and gold? (Wait five seconds)
- Can you remember how your body feels just before you fall asleep? (Wait five seconds)
- Can you imagine ripples on the surface of a lake? (Wait five seconds)
- Are you able to notice if your body feels heavy or light? (Wait five seconds)
- Can you remember the most beautiful outdoor scene you have ever seen? (Wait five seconds)
- (Repeat or add additional items to suit your needs) When your body is ready let your eyes open.

4. Guided imagery. Especially suited for those who:

a. Have a lower need for control.

b. Think more visually than verbally.

c. Find that distraction helps.

d. Have problems with anxiety.

Guided imagery involves helping yourself think about either imaginary or actual events. The things that you concentrate on are usually chosen to achieve a specific goal, such as increase your comfort level, help you remain calm, or encourage you to think more positively about the future. Imagery exercises are among the most enjoyable relaxation techniques, especially for people who are the most inventive when creating scenes they imagine.

Rather than following a script written by someone else, you will probably want to create your own images. By doing this you will be tailoring your imagery to your own needs. Keep this in mind as you read the sample imagery exercises in this section. It will probably be less helpful to use them word for word than it would be to read them to get an idea of the limitless possibilities for creating your own scripts.

The basic idea is to write about something you would like to imagine. This script can then be recorded on a cassette tape for you to listen to with your eyes closed at a later time. Below is an excerpt from a script that could be used by someone who wanted to relax and control pain. Notice that since this person tends to think "in pictures" it contains vivid visual descriptions of events. Someone else, who finds it easier to imagine sounds, physical sensations such as touch, or even smells, might write a completely different script relying more on these senses.

> *As I sit in my chair looking down the beach close to my home, I notice that my body becomes warm, comfortable, and relaxed. I feel these sensations even more as I watch the sun setting, very slowly. It will soon seem to disappear into the ocean. The seagulls flying overhead are gently dipping low to pick up bits of food. As I see this, I notice how comfortable and relaxed my body is becoming. I'm totally involved in watching these things around me. And as I lie here longer and longer, I notice that it is gradually*

getting darker and it becomes harder to see those things that are farther in the distance.... And now that the sun gets lower and lower on the horizon, I appreciate even more the warm, comfortable, relaxed feeling that comes over my body. The beautiful pastel colors of the sunset seem to surround me....

Many people could find that this script, tape recorded with pauses between most of the sentences, would help them become lost in a world of images. It would distract them from their pain and bring their thoughts to more pleasant things. Other people use imagery for completely different purposes. Consider the following dialogue, designed to help one man feel more confident about his ability to cope with his upcoming surgery.

I notice that as I see myself walking around the room I think about many things I have done during my lifetime. I remember graduating from school, getting my driver's license, and going into the service. My family often comes to mind, and I think about all the good and difficult times we have faced together. And as I think of these things I remember that my surgery will begin in just a few hours. As I have done so many times in the past, I talk to my friends and family about my concerns about what could happen. I'm careful to be sure that my imagination does not get out of hand and make me worry about things that are not likely to actually occur. My breathing exercises are working well and I know they are helping me to relax and feel calm and comfortable. My surgeon is in my room now, smiling confidently and telling me that she expects things to go very well in the operating room. As I say good-bye to my family I am wheeled down the hall to the operating room. I continue to practice my breathing, very slowly and deliberately. I fall asleep. I wake up, and now the surgery is over. I look around and see many faces of people who are helping me to feel as comfortable as possible. Although there is some pain, I continue to practice my breathing and keep calm. I know I am coping well with this ordeal and that the anxiety I feel is normal....

Many people find that they need to listen to these tapes only a few times before they begin to notice some improvement in their physical comfort or emotional states. Eventually, many no longer need to rely on the tape recordings and can lead themselves through the imagery just by closing their eyes and thinking.

It may be helpful if you play soft music while you are practicing imagery. Also, remember it's normal for your thoughts to wander during these exercises. If you find you start thinking about things other than your imagery, don't worry. Instead, just bring your thoughts back to the imagery when you can.

5. Hypnosis. Especially suited for those who:

a. Have a lower need for control.
b. Think more visually than verbally.
c. Are looking for a way to control pain or other physical discomfort.

Hypnosis is not the mysterious hocus-pocus some people believe it to be. Actually, it's very much like the guided imagery and sensory awareness described above. With hypnosis people may "see" something they are imagining as clearly as if it actually were happening. This is similar to finding yourself lost in a daydream or becoming emotionally involved with the story in a motion picture, two common occurrences for many of us.

Hypnotized people usually find that their perceptions of the world change. Reality is what is suggested, not necessarily what actually exists. If your hypnotist suggests that the sky is orange you may actually see orange when you look up. If your hypnotist tells you that your pain has turned into a tingling sensation that is what you may feel. Hypnosis is sometimes so effective in changing peoples' perceptions of pain that it occasionally has been used as anesthesia during surgery. People have had operations such as hip replacements, cesarean sections, and heart surgery using nothing but hypnosis to control pain. In these cases it was obviously a very effective method of changing their perceptions of their own discomfort. Although there are many theories, nobody knows how hypnosis works. But we don't really need to know what makes it effective, only that it helps people.

Hypnosis is not for everyone. Perhaps less than 10% of the general population for example, would be able to use hypnosis as the only form of anesthesia during surgery. More than half of us, though, can use it to reduce or even eliminate less severe pain from things such as headaches, medical procedures like spinal taps and back problems. Others find that it helps them to control nausea or anxiety. So, although not everyone can benefit from learning hypnosis, it certainly does provide many people with relief.

The major drawback of hypnosis perhaps is that it should be taught by a very knowledgeable and experienced caregiver. Inexperienced therapists, attempting to try their hand at hypnosis, will probably fail or even cause problems. Therefore, if you are interested in learning hypnotic techniques you should find a practitioner who has experience using hypnosis with other people having your particular problem. This almost always works better than teaching it to yourself out of a book or from cassette tapes that are available in book stores.

Unfortunately, the field of hypnosis seems to have more than its share of quacks. In most states anyone can legally be called a "hypnotist" and still have absolutely no formal education or training. So be sure to pay special attention to credentials when you select someone to teach you hypnosis. Below is a list of signs that might alert you to charlatans practicing in this field.

1. Claims to cure everything from baldness to small breasts (Yes, some clinicians have offered to perform breast enlargement by hypnosis).
2. Fancy sounding degrees not awarded by universities.
3. Caregivers who only have experience doing hypnosis and are not familiar with other forms of treatment. Caregivers with only a few skills are less likely to be effective. Instead, you should be looking for someone who can use hypnosis along with a variety of other techniques to help you with your difficulties.
4. Caregivers who don't seem to have much experience working with other professionals in the community. Again, it is important for every caregiver to know about other practitioners who may be able to help you with different

treatments.

5. People who will perform hypnosis without first interviewing you to be sure hypnosis will be a safe technique for you to use. Problems are fairly rare, but some people have been hurt by the reckless use of hypnosis. Those who are especially likely to suffer include people who have an especially high need for control. Occasionally they will notice an increase in their anxiety level when hypnotized. Others may remember unpleasant or frightening events that happened years earlier. And, very rarely, some people develop more serious psychological problems.
6. Anyone who does hypnosis for entertainment in a bar or high school.

Also, if you are using hypnosis to mask physical symptoms such as pain, difficulty breathing, or stomach upset, you should be aware that you might be "covering up" problems that your caregiver should know about. Some people with chest pain, for example, have used hypnosis to "cure" their discomfort. Because they actually may notice no pain, the problems that caused the pain (such as heart disease) may go untreated.

6. Biofeedback.

Especially suited for those who:

a. Have problems with tight muscles in the back, neck, and shoulders. This may contribute to headache or backache.
b. Like to be able to measure their progress easily.

Biofeedback is a technique that many people use to reduce their muscle tension, pain, and anxiety. Essentially, biofeedback is a way to get information about your body. This is just like what happens when you have your blood pressure taken. With biofeedback though, instead of learning about your blood pressure you learn about how tense or relaxed your muscles are, how fast your heart is beating, how much you are perspiring, or about your temperature. Each of these things tells you something about your level of anxiety and tension.

To learn biofeedback, you first might want to go to a caregiver experienced using it for people having difficulties like yours.

Although many of these practitioners are psychologists, there are other therapists who are also skilled using biofeedback equipment. These people can be social workers, psychotherapists, or other types of biofeedback technicians.

If you find biofeedback helpful you may even decide to purchase some equipment of your own. To get a good idea of the different kinds of biofeedback equipment that are available try contacting the Association for Applied Psychophysiology and Biofeedback in Wheat Ridge Colorado 303–422–8436. They publish a magazine that contains advertisements from many of the major biofeedback companies. Each usually gives brief descriptions of the equipment along with photographs and sometimes price ranges. The magazine also has a number of interesting articles that could be helpful to someone learning about the many uses of biofeedback.

Generally, when you practice biofeedback you will first go to a quiet place and lie down. Then you or your caregiver will put sensors on your body. This may involve using tape, paste, or Velcro to temporarily attach them to your skin. These sensors are usually designed to measure muscle tightness, heart rate, or perspiration. The general idea is that the biofeedback equipment lets you know when any of these things change. So, if your equipment measures muscle tension it would give you a signal, often in the form of a beep, a buzz, or a different number displayed on a screen when you become more tense. The signal gives you concrete information about what your body is doing.

Using this equipment you should be able to measure how well your relaxation strategies are working. To do this, you might first practice two relaxation exercises that seem to work well. Let's say you have chosen diaphragmatic breathing and imagery. You can then practice each of them while you use the biofeedback equipment. The equipment should tell you exactly how well you were able to relax using each of the exercises. In other words, you can use the equipment to see which relaxation strategy works best. Many people, in fact, are quite surprised by the results of the biofeedback equipment. While they may notice no difference in how well different relaxation strategies work, the biofeedback equipment may clearly show that one technique is superior to the other.

7. Active rehearsal

Especially suited for those who:

a. Anticipate a painful or frightening medical procedure.

Perhaps one of the medical procedures for which people rehearse most frequently is childbirth. Many people take classes in the Lamaze (1970) method in the months before delivery to increase their enjoyment of the birth process. In these classes they learn what sensations and sights to expect during childbirth. They also are taught breathing strategies and a variety of techniques designed to prevent them from concentrating on their pain. Sometimes a part of this rehearsal actually involves simulating the pain of contractions. To do this, the woman's "labor coach" may squeeze a part of her body, such as an arm or leg. The woman practices using her pain control techniques while feeling the discomfort caused by the squeeze. Not surprisingly, the Lamaze method has been shown to help women reduce both their pain and their fear during active labor (Leventhal, Leventhal, Shacham, & Easterling, 1989).

People other than pregnant women have practiced for medical tests or treatments. Some rehearse before they have images taken of their bodies with Magnetic Resonance Imagers (MRI). Usually people are required to wear hospital gowns (which sometimes open in the back) during MRI tests. Then they are placed on a tray that slides on a track into a hole through the MRI machine. The machine itself looks like a gigantic clothes dryer. The hole people are slid into resembles the opening in a dryer door. A cage may be clamped around the head to fasten it to the tray and keep it from moving. Other parts of the body can also be restrained in some way, such as by taping the ankles together. Next, all the technicians leave the room. The tray on which the person is lying is then moved through the hole in the MRI. After this, the person is in a small compartment inside the MRI that usually feels about the size of a coffin. During much of the 45 minute test loud noises are heard that make it sound as if someone were operating a lawn mower inside the room.

Not surprisingly, this test frightens many people. One of the ways to rehearse for the MRI is to imagine going through the procedure. To accomplish this, some people first recline on their bed, sofa, or easy chair, and picture as clearly as they can, each of the steps needed to prepare them for the test. Then they may imagine they are being moved into the MRI and that they can hear the loud noises around them. While thinking about these things, it is very important that they also rehearse "coping statements" to help them reduce their own anxiety. The goal is that once they are able to practice saying these coping statements in their rooms they will have an easier time saying them when they are actually taking the test. Here are some examples of the helpful things that people often say to help themselves:

- It's normal to feel some anxiety during this test.
- I don't have to be perfectly relaxed.
- This is a safe test.
- I can stop this test whenever I want.
- I can distract myself by thinking about....
- I will probably be able to get through this test by using my relaxation techniques that I practiced earlier in my room.
- I could rehearse my guided imagery and pretend I'm lying on a noisy tanning bed.

Notice that some of these help people remember that a certain amount of anxiety is normal. In other words, they discourage people from becoming anxious about not being perfectly relaxed. Other statements emphasize that they are safe and can decide to stop the test at any time. Finally, some things people say to themselves remind them that they have many tools to reduce their own anxiety. What's especially nice about rehearsal is that it usually does not require the help of someone else. It can also be done just about any time a quiet room can be found. Although it often helps to be able to see the machinery (or medical procedure) you are afraid of ahead of time, this is usually not essential.

Practice your active rehearsal as often as you feel the need. Some people do it many times, while others find that once or twice is enough.

8. TENS. Especially suited for those who:

a. Have pain for a long time.

TENS, which stands for "transcutaneous electrical nerve stimulation" is a technique by which low-voltage electrical stimulation is applied to an area of the body. This is made possible by using a "TENS unit," which is a battery powered box about the size of a T.V. remote control. This box emits electrical impulses through wires that are temporarily taped to the skin near the area of discomfort. It's believed that TENS works not by distracting people's attention from their pain, but rather by interfering with the transmission of pain signals to the brain. Because the TENS unit does not interfere with most activities, the user typically wears it throughout the day. TENS units have been used to treat pain such as chronic lower back pain, migraine, arthritis, and cancer pain as well as acute discomfort resulting from broken ribs, surgical pain, and even tennis elbow. Although not recommended for people with pacemakers, it's generally a safe procedure that doesn't present the risk of addiction as do many medications.

One of the great advantages of TENS units is that the users are able to adjust the intensity of the stimulation. On days when the pain is the greatest, they simply turn up the voltage for extra relief. Not only might this reduce pain more effectively, but it also often gives people much more control over their treatments.

9. Dogs, rub-downs, and all else. Especially suited for:

a. Everyone!

Set your imagination loose to think of things that will help you relax. Make a list of the twenty things that are likely to help. You may decide that your first choice would be to have your pet brought to your room. Although this was unheard of in the past, some hospitals now allow dogs, cats, and other animals to visit. This is largely because it has been shown that animals may lower their owner's blood pressure, help them relax, and fight loneliness. What a wonderful boost it is for some isolated people to suddenly have a visit from their pet, who may have been their closest companion for years.

The major concern of some hospital administrators is, of

course, that bringing pets into a hospital will be unsanitary. Other times, it's simply one of those rules made by bureaucrats with no reason other than to make life easier for staff. If there is no medical reason that animals cannot be brought to your room, you might insist that you be allowed to have your pet brought to your bedside. Portable travel kennels for airplanes work well for this and should prevent your pet from getting loose in the hallway.

A broad range of needs can be addressed during your hospital stay. For example, another idea is to have your lover ask when the best time would be to put a "Do Not Disturb" sign on your hospital room door. Your practitioners should plan meals, medical tests, and so forth around your interlude. You may even want to ask the nurse to show you how to safely be in bed with your partner without disturbing any medical equipment to which you might be attached. A nurse or another caregiver can also tell you whether or not it is safe for you to be in bed with someone else.

Actually, many kinds of touch are just what people often need to reduce anxiety and pain during long hospital stays. It's often not necessary to have intercourse to get this contact. You may want to have someone brush or wash your hair. Some people find that massage works the best. A few hospitals even offer massage therapy. If your hospital doesn't, you could have a friend or even a professional massage therapist come to your room.

Other ideas are to take up a hobby, play card games, read, or even put on video tapes of your favorite movies. A portable compact disc player or a tape recorder with headphones might give you the chance to listen to your favorite music without disturbing others. And, in case you haven't noticed, your home V.C.R. will probably hook up easily to your hospital room T.V.

Other Benefits

Some studies have suggested that relaxation techniques along with information about what to expect during treatment may benefit people with medical problems in ways other than just increasing comfort. One review (Devine and Cook, 1983) of 49 scientific studies concluded that hospitalized people who: a) knew what a test or surgery would feel like, b) learned exercises to reduce anxiety or prevent other complications, and/or c) had more emotional support from caregivers or friends and relatives spent one and one-third fewer days in the hospital. In other words, informed consumers who knew how to relax and/or had support from others tended to leave the hospital earlier.

Another investigator (Anderson, 1987) looked at people who were preparing for heart surgery. He found that many benefitted from knowing what to expect before and after their surgeries and by learning exercises to help themselves turn in bed, breathe deeply, and prevent muscle stiffness. After surgery they showed less emotional distress, had better physical recoveries, and fewer problems with high blood pressure.

Logically, some writers have stressed the importance of teaching people both what will happen to them and what their medical tests and treatments will feel like (Suls and Wan, 1989). This information may help them for its reassurances that the sensations they are experiencing are normal and that things are going smoothly. Not surprisingly, those who are prepared in these ways often report less pain and better moods. Of course, one implication of this is that the reader should insist on learning not only what will be done but what it will feel like. Will the test hurt? And, if so, how much and for how long? Don't just accept vague statements that it will hurt "a little." You might also want to see a picture of what will be done. Another option is to ask to look any equipment that will be used in your treatment.

Control Your Pain-Fighting Medication

Many people who have severe pain from surgery, illness, or injury receive injections of powerful pain-killing medications. Until recently, they had to wait for their physicians or nurses to give them each dose of these pain-killers. Unfortunately, some people suffer for hours before their busy caregivers have time to attend to their needs. And, when the injections are finally given, large doses are often needed to control the pain which has gradually become quite severe. These large doses sometimes cause other side effects such as sleepiness, nausea, or even breathing difficulties.

During the past few years there has been an alternative for many people suffering from pain. It's called "Patient Controlled Analgesia" or, in short, PCA. It lets people give themselves injections of pain-fighting medication when they need it. PCA equipment consists of a pump that stands by the bedside. When a button is pushed, it delivers medication through a tube to a needle that is usually inserted into an arm. With this equipment, whenever you feel pain you simply push the button and the pump will deliver a small dose of medication into your bloodstream. There are even safeguards on the pump that prevent you from giving yourself too much medication.

This new technology makes it possible for people to have many smaller, usually safer, injections the instant they are needed. It also helps people use less medication. For example, no medication will be taken when people are asleep or when they have less discomfort. Perhaps one of the most important benefits, though, is that it gives people a sense of having some control over their care. They no longer have to rely on others to give them medicine and therefore they have more power. This can be very reassuring to those who dread waiting for their caregivers to respond to their requests for medication.

Your practitioner will be able to tell you if it would be possible to use PCA for your pain. If you anticipate needing surgery or any other painful procedure, be sure to ask about PCA well in advance. Otherwise you may have to wait for a long time for your caregivers to set up the equipment, which may be hidden in a distant corner of the hospital.

Even if you don't use PCA, whenever possible, be sure to discuss all methods of pain control with your practitioner long before you will need them. If you do this you should be able to develop a pain control plan before it is needed. Not only may this calm your fears but it could prevent long and uncomfortable delays in your treatment.

Occasionally people notice that their caregivers are somewhat reluctant to use medication to help them control pain. But in reality, there may be no compelling medical reason why painkillers should not be used. Occasionally, this reluctance to prescribe pain medication occurs when a caregiver suspects that a customer abuses drugs or alcohol. One concern, that they will seldom state out loud, is that giving you more medication will only increase your chances of addiction. He may also be afraid that the pain-killers would react adversely with whatever drugs he fears are already in your system.

A long-haired friend of mine accidentally gashed his arm when installing some windows. He went to the emergency room of a nearby hospital dressed in his dirty work clothes. Once there, they cleaned his wounds and gave him over thirty stitches, all without one drop of medication to control his pain. Although the emergency room personnel wouldn't say it, he suspected that their refusal to ease his discomfort was related to his appearance.

If you think that your caregiver is withholding medication from you for similar reasons, your only option might be to deal with the problem directly. First, it's possible that your caregiver hasn't even asked you about your drug use but instead assumes you're hooked on something. If this is the case bring up the subject yourself. If you don't take drugs, state that clearly and say that see no reason why it would be harmful to give you more medication to control your pain. You might even insist that the caregiver check your "references" by contacting other practitioners who have treated you in the past. If there is reason your caregiver should be concerned about your drug use though, again, for your own good, be sure to let him or her know.

Pitfalls For Those Who Are Fighting Pain

If you have pain that lasts for a long time, you may notice that it eventually brings some rewards. This is often the case with problems like chronic back pain where people feel more uncomfortable when they do strenuous physical activities. Now, you might have an excuse not to work as many hours at that boring job you planned to quit in a few years anyway. Your spouse might take on extra jobs around that house that you can't do such as mow the lawn, do the laundry, or bathe the dog. If you are lucky, you might even get other goodies like back rubs and your favorite meals.

Don't feel guilty for accepting these favors. You probably

need many of them. They make it easier for you to get through the day in spite of your pain. There is a danger, however, if you start getting used to having someone do things for you that you can actually do for yourself. You might learn to sit on the couch most of the day while your spouse takes on all of the child care responsibilities, even the easy ones. Some people learn to delegate jobs to their kids. One result of these new habits is that the person with pain becomes more inactive. They can easily gain weight and lose muscle tone. Unfortunately, this physical "deconditioning" usually causes an increase in pain because weakened muscles can often not hold ones' body in the most comfortable position.

Assuming there is no medical reason for your inactivity, you may be able to prevent your pain from getting worse by staying in good physical shape. This doesn't just mean following an exercise program. It also means making sure that you continue to do all those odd jobs during the rest of the day. Watch for the little things you may be tempted to do more often like asking family members to get up at the dinner table to refill your glass. If you can, mow your own lawn instead of hiring the kid next door. These jobs add up and may make you much more physically fit if you do them yourself. They also have the positive effect of increasing self-esteem and self-confidence.

Another pitfall of getting favors when you are in pain is that the favors may actually encourage you to complain more. For example, a woman may get in the habit of rubbing her husband's back when he groans in pain. Eventually, because of her eagerness to help, he may groan whenever he has even a little discomfort. What happens is that the back rubs encourage him to complain. Don't misunderstand though. Back rubs and other favors are fine. Just be sure they don't contribute to your problem. To help prevent this from happening, reward yourself when you are more active physically or talk less about your discomfort. For a day of hard work you could go to a movie or out to dinner. Be generous and creative with these rewards. Just be sure that you earn them for being more, not less, energetic.

If you enjoy back rubs or other favors you might also make them a normal part of your relationship, not just something that happens when you are in pain. In this arrangement you won't need to show your pain in order to be touched or have your favorite meal. Not only could these changes improve your relationship, but they might take away dangerous "rewards" for complaining about your discomfort.

You might also need to pay attention to personality traits that cause you to be less active and to complain. Some people are rather passive and have difficulty making their own decisions. Quite often they depend on others to make those choices for them. In fact, they seem to almost enjoy letting others take charge of their lives. Imagine what happens when they develop a problem with chronic pain. They suddenly see themselves as having a legitimate reason to rely on others even more. After all, with their chronic pain they have an excuse to assume less responsibility for working hard and directing their own lives. They do less and less and eventually end up depressed and in poor physical shape.

Perhaps you won't recognize these personality traits in yourself. If you do, though, you may need to learn to be more assertive and self-reliant. This will probably be a difficult job, especially since it will mean that you should change habits that you have acquired over a lifetime. You will need to learn to do things for yourself, make your own decisions, and rely on other people less. Although it will probably be uncomfortable for you to do this early on, eventually you might be much happier with your life. You could also read either *Your Perfect Right* (Alberti & Emmons, 1988) or *Self-Assertion for Women* (Butler, 1981). These books are written to help people learn to control and direct their lives in ways that will not interfere with the rights of others.

CHAPTER 7

Helping to Heal Yourself

"I can't express anger, that's one of the problems I have. I grow a tumor instead."
–Woody Allen (**Manhattan*****, 1979)***

Many scientists are beginning to explore the ways that our moods, thoughts, and emotions affect our physical health. Partly as a result of this movement many writers have attributed everything from cancer to hair loss to psychological states. While some of these claims have been supported by scientific research, others have been based on half-truths or apparently on the imaginations of the writers. The "treatments" presented in their books and articles may be particularly attractive to consumers who are frantically looking for cures. In some cases their judgment is so clouded by desperation they are willing to try almost anything.

Treatments that encourage people to cure themselves by changing their thoughts or emotions can be among the most tempting of these therapies. Not only may they seem to provide legitimate reasons for illness, but they also promise that people can actually do something about their problems. This may make the consumer feel much less helpless. It's also likely that people are attracted to unproven therapies because they emphasize curing and caring for oneself, something highly valued in modern society (Cassileth, 1989). Today, many of us find ourselves encouraged to take more and more responsibility for ourselves. As a whole, we exercise more, eat better, and shop more carefully for health care. Certainly, treatments that promise to help us take even better care of ourselves can be tempting.

Cancer

Some of these questionable treatments are designed for the person fighting cancer. In part, they are based on scientific studies of the immune systems of laboratory animals. The immune systems of both animals and people protect the body from foreign substances called "antigens." These include bacteria, physical objects such as splinters or rusty nails, and even some cancers. Immune systems work by releasing special cells, referred to as "antibodies," into the bloodstream. Each of these antibodies recognizes and attacks specific antigens. At least as early as the 1950s, it was known that mice that were put in stressful situations, such as overcrowded cages, soon were less able to fight off certain diseases. Apparently this occurred because their immune systems produced fewer antibodies. These studies have been repeated many times through the years and have given scientists some fascinating and useful information on how immune systems work.

Later research on animals, however, has shown that some stress may actually improve animals' ability to ward off disease. Whether or not stress impairs or helps organisms' immune system has been shown to be related to a number of things, including the sex of the animal, the intensity and kind of stress, and the type of antigen being studied. So it appears that we can't say simply that a decrease in stress causes a stronger immune system. Sometimes it's the other way around. Scientists are only beginning to understand this complex process and know more about the ways emotions effect animals' ability to fight off disease.

Other studies have looked at the effects of stress on human immune system functioning. In one of these (Schleifer, et al., 1983) the authors looked at changes in the immune systems of men whose wives were treated for, and eventually died from, breast cancer. The scientists found that the men's immune systems produced fewer disease-fighting cells during the first two months after their wives' deaths. It also seemed likely that the long term stress of having a sick wife may have caused even more problems with immune functioning than would have stress that lasted a shorter period of time.

One researcher (Adler, 1989) found that men were more likely to have diseases if their wives had died. Interestingly, women whose husbands die do not seem to show these same problems. It has been speculated that the death of a spouse may not affect women in the same way because they receive more emotional support from others or somehow cope with bereavement more effectively than men.

Another study (Spiegel, Bloom, Kraemer & Gottheil, 1989) looked at the long term survival of a large group of women with breast cancer. The researchers led psychotherapy groups for some of the women. During the group sessions women were encouraged to talk about their cancer and the affect it had on their lives. They also discussed some of the physical effects of their treatments and were taught hypnosis for pain control. Many were shown how to be more assertive with their physicians and to fight social isolation by developing stronger emotional ties with other group members. Ten years after the start of the project, the researchers found that those women who were in therapy groups lived twice as long as those who had no therapy. The authors guessed that the social support of being in therapy somehow helped the women cope more effectively with stress. Conceivably, this may have helped them live longer by strengthening their immune systems. They also speculated that the group may have helped the women to live longer by teaching them to comply with treatment more or by encouraging them to have better diets or exercise habits. For example, people who were able to reduce their pain with hypnosis may have had an easier time sticking to exercise routines.

Even though the results of this study were encouraging, it's important to remember that the authors still could not show exactly what made the women who received group therapy live longer. The results may even have been due to chance. If this was the case, the next researcher studying the same thing would probably find that the group therapy had no effect on survival time. These problems highlight the fact that this research is still in its infancy. There is, as of now, no psychotherapy that has been proven to help people with cancer live longer.

Although the research is still in a primitive state, some authors (Simonton & Simonton, 1978, Siegel 1986) have written books teaching people how to "treat" their cancer with imagery. For example, people with cancer may be encouraged to visualize their bodies fighting cancerous tumors. Then, they may be told to try to see their immune systems attacking the cancer. Their immune systems may suddenly become an army of warriors furiously attacking the invading tumors. Eventually their immune systems are victorious in this struggle as the tumor is "destroyed" and removed from the body.

One major goal of this imagery is to strengthen the immune system. The rationale for this comes largely from the types of studies described above, where functioning of immune systems has been shown to be related to emotional states. The main question in the minds of many continues to be "Is there sufficient evidence to conclude that imagery helps people with cancer?" The answer to this is "no." As yet, there are no conclusive scientific studies showing that people can use imagery to cure their cancer.

But this shouldn't discourage everyone from using these techniques. First, these methods may be effective. In fact there is some evidence that suggests that they could help. They also probably won't hurt, providing that people don't decide to use imagery instead of proven cancer treatments. And finally, they may give people a much needed sense of control and power over their disease. This could greatly improve their mood and give them the encouragement they need to fight on. In other words, a sense of control is important in emotional adjustment. The important thing is for consumers to shop carefully and not blindly subject themselves to treatments with unknown risks and benefits. In this case imagery for cancer is fine, provided that it is not claimed to be a cure-all.

There are many other health problems that have been effectively treated using both medical and psychological techniques. With some of these illnesses, in fact, it's essential to look at behaviors that cause the problems, make them worse, or prevent them from going away. Again, this means that the consumer must be involved and must not rely on others to do it all. Consumers may need to make drastic changes in their lives as well as to learn relaxation or stress management skills. Without them, medical treatment alone may be of little use. Remember also that this book was written by a psychologist, with little training in other specialty areas that may offer solutions. These include dietetics, chiropractic, and pharmacy, to name a few. It is your responsibility to ask these and other professionals for treatments that may be of help to you. One particularly good source of information may be the National Cancer Institute. They have a toll-free cancer information service that you can call. The telephone number is 800–422–6237.

Heart Disease

Today it's common for people to believe that behavior and mood can affect their heart. "Type A" behavior, as it has come to be known, is one personality style that has been thought to contribute to heart disease (Rosenman & Brand, 1975). People who show Type A traits are those who are described as competitive and angry. In particular, they usually think they are behind schedule and feel a need to finish projects ahead of time. Type B people, in contrast, are seen as more relaxed and laid back. They don't share Type A's intense desire to conquer the world and may prefer to be much less competitive.

It is thought that some people with Type A personalities may suffer from a variety of physical problems because of long term chemical changes in the body. These difficulties include hardening of the arteries, high blood pressure, problems with circulation, and congestive heart failure. Although the research is not at all conclusive, there is some evidence that people who are most likely to experience these problems are those Type A's who are the most angry and hostile.

If you see these traits in yourself, you may want to change your behavior and reduce your overall stress. People who have learned to manage their stress more effectively have reduced their probability of early death (Rahe, Ward, & Hayes, 1979) and of heart attacks (Powell, Friedman, & Thoresen, 1984). This stress management may be done with a variety of methods. They include relaxation training (described in chapter six), counseling, exercise, and sometimes drugs. The counseling usually focuses on helping people look at the causes of their over-active lifestyles and helps them to learn to behave more calmly and less aggressively.

Those who are interested in reading about these treatments might turn to *Stress, Sanity, & Survival* (Woolfolk & Richardson, 1978) for ideas on how to lead a slower and more balanced life.

Another book is *Treating Type A Behavior and Your Heart* (Friedman & Ulmer, 1984).

Breathing

It's common for people with physical problems to have trouble breathing. Of course, if you can't breathe correctly, you should always have a physical exam. This will determine whether or not something dangerous is causing your difficulties.

Sensations of breathlessness and hyperventilation are two breathing problems that often have both physical and psychological causes. Both are found in people who are in poor physical condition and also feeling anxious. A common scenario is for someone with heart or lung problems to feel as if it's hard to get a full breath of air. In the beginning, this is often almost totally due to physical causes. Soon, the person concentrates more on the discomfort in the lungs and chest. Anxiety increases and the person begins to feel frightened. Although reassurance by caregivers helps, thoughts such as "They don't know I won't stop breathing" and "If I don't concentrate on each breath I might die" are common. The anxiety, in turn, can cause abdominal muscles to tighten, eventually causing even more problems breathing. What happens then, is that breathing problems originally caused by physical problems are made much worse by anxiety and fear.

A good example of this occurs with some people who have had lung transplants. Because of disease, these people have had both of their lungs replaced by the lungs of a donor. One of the problems with a new set of lungs is that the nerves coming from the original lungs have been destroyed during surgery. Once transplanted, the person no longer feels the sensations from the lungs that used to signal that a full breath had been taken. Instead, while they may actually be filling up their lungs with each breath, they feel as if they are short of breath. Understandably this can lead to anxiety, sleep loss, and muscle tension. These problems, in turn, can further interfere with breathing.

If you are having breathlessness or are feeling as if you are not getting a full breath of air, there are a number of things you might do which are meant to help you regain the trust and confidence in your body that you may have lost due to illness. They can also help you strengthen the muscles that control your breathing. To begin, you may want to contact a caregiver such as a respiratory therapist, dance/movement therapist, or yoga instructor to help you learn to breathe deeply. These caregivers often work in hospitals and many other facilities. It is likely that they will teach you how to do diaphragmatic breathing (see page 163) or other breathing techniques, depending on your needs.

The next important step in recovery is to look at the issue of control. When people have difficulty breathing they often pay close attention to each breath, trying to control exactly how long each lasts, how deep each one is, and so forth. While some attempts to control your breathing are fine, be careful that you don't go overboard. This is because when you think about your breathing too much you are really telling yourself that your body is not to be trusted and needs to be watched. Obviously this is no way to build confidence.

A better strategy is usually to practice giving up control, bit by bit. Because this may be just the opposite of what you feel comfortable doing, it may at first be frightening. There are ways to do this relatively comfortably, however. First, you might begin by giving up control of just one breath. Let your body take a breath "on its own." As you do this watch how your chest and lungs seem to take over, with no direction from you. Eventually you should be able to let your body take two consecutive breaths, then three, and then more. It's likely that after a while you will feel more comfortable with your breathing and have more confidence in your body.

Another tactic is distraction. This is most often done by people who have problems taking deep breaths. With distraction, you might decide to try to think about a T.V. show, your visitors, or whatever else holds your interest. This could help you gradually think about your body less and feel less of a need to measure every breath. Perhaps the major problem with distraction is that some people do it thinking they are trying to get their minds off dangerous physical symptoms. When they do think about their breathing, it's still frightening because they haven't learned that the symptoms, in many cases, are harmless. So if you do distract yourself, keep in mind that another goal should be to remember that the symptoms may not be dangerous.

Hyperventilation occurs in people who have problems with anxiety. When they hyperventilate, they breathe too quickly and too deeply. Sometimes this causes them to feel lightheaded and even to faint. A simple solution for hyperventilation is to breathe slowly through the nose. This should reduce the amount of extra oxygen going into your bloodstream and prevent you from feeling lightheaded.

Stomach And Digestive Problems

Your stomach, intestines, and bowels are some of the body organs most sensitive to emotional upset and stress. Common symptoms include abdominal cramps, diarrhea, constipation, difficulty eating certain foods, nausea, and vomiting. In fact, you may notice that these symptoms get worse during times when the stress in your life is most severe. This doesn't mean though that your problems are all "in your head." Instead, it suggests that if you do have actual physical problems, their symptoms are made worse by stress.

Stress management techniques are often quite helpful in treating stomach and digestive symptoms. Chapter six describes a number of these techniques to promote relaxation and fight stress. Keep in mind, though, that just because your symptoms get better when you relax doesn't mean that you can ignore any true physical problems. Always be sure to get any necessary medical treatment and don't just rely on stress management skills. And of course, be sure that your caregivers know you are using relaxation techniques to help control your symptoms.

Dieticians are also often very helpful to some people with these problems. Sometimes they recommend special foods that don't cause nausea or are easier to digest. They also might suggest that you avoid certain types of food, such as proteins and solid foods, that sometimes cause nausea.

Sleep

There are many reasons, both physical and psychological, that people have difficulty sleeping. Sleep researchers are just beginning to understand what happens when we sleep, and how this can be disrupted by physical problems, medications, or emotional states. Below are descriptions of a few of the most common sleep disorders and their treatment. If you have persistent problems with sleep, be sure to see a caregiver experienced in the diagnosis and treatment of sleep problems. Preferably, the person works with people such as physicians, psychologists, nurses, and technicians who are able to treat both the physical and emotional aspects of your problem. Also, you will notice that there are often things that you can do to help yourself with many of these sleep difficulties, even if they do have a physical cause. For more information a good resource is the publication *The Sleep Disorders* (Hauri, 1982).

Feeling sleepy during the day even though you sleep all night.

A physical problem called "sleep apnea" often causes people to feel sleepy during the day. People who have sleep apnea stop breathing at night for periods lasting as long as two minutes. After this, the sleeping person may gasp for air and then breathe normally again for a short while. This cycle can repeat hundreds of times through the night. Sleep apnea seems to make it impossible for people to remain in a deep sleep and feel rested in the morning. Sometimes it even causes heart problems, probably because it prevents the heart from receiving enough oxygen.

There are a number of medical treatments for sleep apnea. Medication is often used as well as machines to pump air into the sleeping person's lungs throughout the night. Both of these treatments can produce dramatic improvement in a short time. Also, surgery is used in some cases to widen the airway in the back of the throat or to create a "breathing hole" in the neck that is opened at night.

In addition to these medical treatments, some people find that they can control their sleep apnea by sleeping on their sides or stomachs. This greatly reduces the number of times people with one type of sleep apnea (called "positional sleep apnea") stop breathing. It is likely this treatment works because the flaps in their throats are held open when they are in these new positions. If your caregiver suggests that you learn to sleep on your stomach or side, try this: first get out a needle and thread along with an old tightly fitting t-shirt. Sew four or five small pockets in the middle of the back of the shirt. They should be evenly spaced so they are over your spine, running from just below the collar to the shirt's lower hem. Put one tennis ball in each of the pockets and you are ready for bed. Unless you sleep on your stomach or side you will be poked in the back by at least one tennis ball. Some people can train themselves to sleep on their sides by propping pillows around themselves in bed. Often overweight people find that their sleep apnea improves when they lose weight. This is because the extra fat in and around the neck seems to interfere with breathing.

Can't fall asleep at bedtime

Perhaps the most common sleep complaint is difficulty falling asleep. While it takes most people less than 20 minutes to fall asleep others toss and turn for hours. Caffeine and some prescription medications are frequent physical causes of these difficulties. If you are in the hospital, the constant beeps and clicks from machines as well as the 24 hour a day presence of nurses might also keep you awake. You may need to ask for some things to be turned off at night, to have your door closed, or for earplugs.

If you have trouble falling asleep at home you have probably learned to associate the bed and bedtime with anxiety and stress, rather than with sleep. Perhaps one night long ago you were kept up a little later than usual by your children. You worried that you would not get enough sleep to be at your best the next day at work. Because of this you probably tried to fall asleep quickly. To your surprise you learned that even though you tried to fall asleep you seemed to stay awake longer than usual. In fact the more you tried to sleep the longer you stayed awake. Soon, you found yourself struggling to sleep almost every night before work, hoping that you would get enough rest for the next day. On nights when you didn't have work the following day you didn't try to fall asleep the night before. And, on these nights, you usually dozed off in just a few minutes.

What you learned was that trying to fall asleep usually caused insomnia. It's a paradox. The more you try to sleep the longer you will stay awake. So don't try to hurry or force sleep, just let it sneak up on you on it's own. Also, if you can't fall asleep in 20 minutes or so, get out of bed and watch T.V., balance your checkbook, or get some other work done. Go back to bed only when you are tired. Don't force yourself to stay in bed. The only thing that will do is help you associate the bed with anxiety, tension, and sleeplessness. If this happens you might notice that when you first lie down you feel anxious. Perhaps the muscles in your neck and back tighten in anticipation of your struggle for sleep. This is a signal that you should not be in bed when you are anxious. In fact, about the only activities reserved for the bed should be sleep and sex. Neither (hopefully!) will cause anxiety. Also, keep in mind that you don't need much sleep to do well at work the next day. Although you may feel bad, research has shown that people can do an excellent job at even complicated intellectual tasks after having practically no sleep for days. Also, be sure to keep a regular schedule, going to bed and waking up at a regular time every day. This will help get your body into a pattern where it cues itself to fall asleep at a certain time.

Some people have sleep problems because of excitement. They think about all the interesting things they are involved in during the day and can't seem to turn their minds off at night. While very extreme forms of this are sometimes associated with mental illness, most of the time it happens in people who are too active during the day. They often find that a "wind down" period at night helps them sleep much better. During this time they do things that are calming and don't remind them of whatever causes their excitement, such as projects at work.

A few words about sleep medications. These drugs, referred to as "hypnotics," only work well for a short time, typically from one to four weeks. When you stop taking them after several weeks, you will probably find that you have developed a dependence on them and your sleep will get worse. Also, some medications cause problems with memory, dizziness, and even hallucinations. It's probably not a good idea then to rely on sleeping pills more than three or four nights a month. Of course, always remember your caregiver's instructions when taking any sleep medication.

Some people find that L-tryptophan, a naturally occurring amino acid found in many protein-rich foods, helps them sleep. There is quite a bit of tryptophan for example, in turkey. This is why whole families often fall asleep in the living room like a pride of lions after Thanksgiving meals. Their systems are saturated with tryptophan. To take advantage of this natural sleep aid, you may want to eat some of the following foods just before bedtime.

- Milk
- Cheese (especially cottage and cheddar)
- Eggs
- Soybean flower and nuts
- Poultry
- Red meat

Wake up during the night

Sometimes people can't sleep without waking up several times at night. When morning comes, they are usually tired and not at all refreshed. There are physical problems that cause difficulty sleeping soundly. These include hormonal changes, physical illness, and alcohol use before bedtime. Usually, though, people with this problem have fairly stressful lives. They often have chronic tension or worry. The most effective treatment will usually combine the short term use of hypnotic medications with changes in lifestyle. Here, the person may decide to take a less stressful job, learn relaxation techniques, or have counseling to help them deal with depression or other worries.

Waking up early in the morning

Some people fall asleep quickly at night but then wake up early in the morning. Although they may be exhausted at 3:00 or 4:00 A.M. they find it impossible to get to sleep again. Often this problem happens to people who are depressed. They may feel sad and think there is no hope their lives will improve. While most depression goes away without professional help, many people choose to take prescription medication and/or receive counseling to help change their moods.

Leg twitches

Although most people's legs twitch as they first fall asleep, others, especially older people, have leg movements hundreds of times each night. This jerking seems to interfere with sleep in many people as they wake up feeling not refreshed and tired. There are a variety of known physical causes for this problem and it is generally treated with medication.

Panic Attacks

Panic attacks are a very common problem, especially for people who feel vulnerable or frightened because of physical illness. These attacks feel like sudden bursts of extreme anxiety. They last from a few minutes to several hours. Usually people notice a number of physical symptoms that go along with the panic, including a rapid heartbeat, perspiration, dizziness, and feeling faint. Often there are fears of going crazy, dying, or of losing control. At first these panic attacks may seem to hit unexpectedly. Eventually though, many people notice that they happen when they are out in public, especially when they aren't with a trusted friend. When they are out, they may worry almost constantly about having an attack. After they notice the first signs of panic, usually a rapidly beating heart, their first reaction may be to try to stop the panic. They might try to distract themselves, they could go home or to a place where they feel more secure, or they could take medication. Quite often it's reassuring for them to be with someone else who they trust during the times when they are most likely to panic. This is because the other person is someone who could help in the event of emergency. In fact, some people may not experience any anxiety at all if they are with someone who would help if an anxiety attack occurred.

Occasionally symptoms similar to those of panic attacks are caused by serious physical conditions such as heart disease. Because of this, it's always a good idea to discuss these problems with your caregiver and to have a thorough physical exam. Quite often, though, people will have no health problems and still continue to experience panic.

Panic attacks are a classic example of a problem caused by both physical and psychological problems. There is evidence that some types of panic attacks are inherited. Many people who panic report that a mother, father, or other relative suffers from a similar problem. Also, there is research that shows there are physical differences in the brains of people who suffer from panic attacks. Perhaps not surprisingly then, certain medications have been shown to be remarkably effective in some people who have this problem. Also, people with a heart condition called "mitral valve prolapse" seem to have panic attacks more often than those who do not. It is still unclear, though, exactly how these heart problems could cause such severe anxiety.

But there are also definite psychological causes for panic. Remember that the panic may happen only in certain situations, such as just before an uncomfortable medical test, when driving alone on the freeway, or when in a movie theater or restaurant. There is no physical reason that panic should occur just during these times. Instead, fear triggers the panic. Panic also may become much worse when a person is under chronic stress or feeling vulnerable. This might occur during a messy divorce, a long term physical illness, when moving away from home to college, or even after the death of a friend.

People with panic attacks sometimes believe they are irrationally afraid of going out in public or being in confined places. This belief is usually based on their observation that their panic attacks happen most often in these situations. In fact, this misperception led to the original name for the condition, "agoraphobia," which literally means, "fear of the marketplace." In reality, people aren't afraid of the marketplace. Instead they are frightened of the panic they experience when they go there. This is called "fear of fear" (Chambless & Gracely, 1989; Clark, 1986). It means that people are frightened of the physical sensations they have during panic. This could be out of concern that they will pass out or lose control in public, die alone in their homes from a heart attack, or lose control of their car when on the freeway. Whatever their fear, they usually do everything they can to prevent more attacks from happening.

One irony is that when these people try to control their panic or make it go away, it usually gets worse. Their attempts to control their symptoms usually backfire as trying to "calm down" usually cause even more distress. What they haven't learned is that one way to stop panic is to give up control. In other words, let the panic happen. In fact, some people even try to make the panic worse. To their surprise, most eventually notice that when they don't try to make the panic go away, it usually gets better.

Other techniques for dealing with panic include keeping your mind on your physical symptoms. Don't try to distract yourself because this may give you the message that the panic symptoms are a terribly scary thing that you need to prevent at all cost. Remember, the panic will be unpleasant, but it is very unlikely that it will hurt you. Next, be nice to yourself. Most people who have this problem are very critical of themselves. They tell themselves that they are weak or defective and should be able just to keep a stiff upper lip like everyone else. This generally just makes people even more ashamed of themselves and of their panic. As a result, they may try to fight the panic even more. Instead, it's usually much more helpful to allow yourself to be less than perfect. You will be taking a big step in this direction once you can accept the fact that just because you suffer from panic attacks you aren't a bad person. Again this will help you accept the attacks and avoid fighting the panic when it occurs. Finally, practice going places that have triggered your panic in the past. Do this gradually. At first you may want to venture only to certain stores or on certain roads. Eventually you may find yourself traveling farther away from home to places that you once avoided. When you do have panic give yourself permission to go back home. Don't feel ashamed to give up. You aren't superman and shouldn't expect to make progress every day.

There is quite a bit of good reading material on panic disorders. One book, in particular, entitled *Overcoming Agoraphobia* (Goldstein & Stainback, 1987). You may also decide to join a support group for people with panic attacks. There are many of these nowadays as people are recognizing that this is such a common problem. You could also contact the Anxiety Disorders Association of America at 133 Rollins Avenue, Suite 4B, Rockville, Maryland 20852-4004. The telephone number is 301–231–9350. They might be able to give you the names of support groups or caregivers specializing in treating panic disorders who practice in you location.

Headaches

Headaches are one of the problems caregivers are most often asked to cure. Almost everyone at least occasionally suffers from headache pain, and for some the discomfort is severe. Fortunately, there are many effective treatments for the headache sufferer. Some of these involve medication, which is often the easiest and most effective way to get relief. Other methods depend on the individual to learn relaxation techniques or to make changes in lifestyle or diet. It is these strategies that give the consumer more power and control. By using them, the consumer can often reduce or eliminate the pain without relying on medication.

Headaches can be triggered by many things. Perhaps the most common is psychological stress, something that often causes "muscle contraction" headaches. Typically the person with muscle contraction headaches first notices tightness in the shoulder or neck muscles, often when feeling tense or anxious. This tightness then seems to move up the back of the neck and cause a headache near the base of the skull. Gradually, this pain may move forward around the sides or the top of the head.

"Migraines" are another common form of headache. People with migraines often notice that they tend to occur during relatively calm periods following several days of emotional stress. For example, they might happen more frequently on weekends after a week of stressful work. It is also likely that migraines are to some extent inherited and therefore are partly caused by biological factors. As with so many problems then, it appears that migraines have both physical and psychological causes. Often migraines begin when the person notices changes in vision such as partial blindness, flashes of light, or spots. Occasionally people even notice difficulty speaking or numbness in part of the body before the most severe pain begins. The pain itself is generally worse than a muscle tension headache and is commonly accompanied by nausea and vomiting. It is often felt just behind one eye or on one side of the head.

Some people have headaches caused by purely physical problems. For example, the person with cancer might have pain because of the pressure of a growing tumor within the skull. Others have eye or dental problems that can cause headache pain. Because of the often serious physical problems then that can cause pain the headache sufferer should always be sure to get a thorough physical examination.

Regardless of the original cause of your headaches, it is likely that you can learn to reduce your pain without medication. Below are three basic psychological techniques that are commonly used by headache suffers.

Relaxation training

Different types of relaxation training are the most common psychological treatments for headaches. As described in chapter six, these include diaphragmatic breathing, progressive muscle relaxation, sensory awareness, and biofeedback. The general idea is that each of these strategies helps reduce the muscle tension that contributes to headache pain. By diligently practicing one or more of these techniques, people can often learn to keep their muscles relaxed enough either to prevent headaches from occurring or to make them much less painful.

Relaxation techniques may also be helpful even if muscle tension was not the original cause of the headache. For example, someone whose headaches are triggered by dental problems most likely will find that his or her neck and shoulder muscles tighten in response to discomfort. This tightening, in turn, may make the original headache even more severe. So while the dental problems are the original cause of the pain, the person's response to that pain (muscle tightening) makes the pain worse. It is this added discomfort that can often be helped by learning relaxation training.

Hypnosis

Recall from chapter six that hypnosis can be used to change the way people experience the world. This includes the sensations they feel in their bodies. Hypnosis can sometimes be used to change a person's perceptions of headache pain. For example some people are taught to believe it isn't there, others are shown how to feel as if the pain were instead a tingling sensation, and some are simply told that they will not notice or remember any discomfort.

Hypnosis may be a particularly useful technique for people whose headaches are due primarily to physical problems such as tumors. This is because the main goal usually isn't to reduce muscle tension, but instead to change the way the person experiences pain.

Stress management

People who notice their headaches get much worse when they are under stress often have less pain after they learn how to reduce their overall level of tension. This can be done in many ways. Often the person with headaches will take a less stressful job or buy a smaller and more affordable house. Some people learn to be more assertive and turn down extra work on the job. Others take more vacations, learn how to discipline their children more effectively, or stop abusing drugs or alcohol.

There are more ways to control headaches than taking medicine and using psychological techniques. Some practitioners urge people to avoid certain foods such as coffee, red wine, or chocolate. Each of these has been shown to cause headaches in certain people. Others offer alternatives such as massage therapy or acupuncture. If you need help, be sure to find out what many different caregivers can offer. You may have to do plenty of research in the library or shop around before you find someone with the skills to help you.

Smoking

People who want to stop smoking often feel very much out of control. They may see themselves as slaves to tobacco, a habit they can't seem to break no matter how hard they try. Some look for miracle cures promised by dishonest caregivers or companies that want to push the latest stop-smoking gadget or program. Watch out for them. They often claim that 80 to 90% of their customers stop smoking forever. In fact, even the best stop-smoking programs only help about half of the people stop smoking for a year or more. Usually the result of peoples' participation in these dishonest programs is more frustration and helplessness.

When you decide to stop smoking, you can think about your cigarette use in two different ways. First, you can consider it to be a physical addiction to nicotine. This drug can cause very uncomfortable withdrawal symptoms for the person trying to quit. You can also look at smoking as a bad habit. In this case, it may be something that you do without thinking during times such as social occasions or after meals. It is usually necessary to look at smoking from both of these perspectives in order to develop a plan to help you stop. Both the physical addiction and the bad habit need to be treated. Caregivers or treatments that don't take both of these into account are probably going to fail.

An effective stop smoking plan might first help you with the part of smoking that is a bad habit. In this plan you might be encouraged to pay more attention to times when you "automatically" light up. This could help you think before you have a cigarette. It could also help you identify things that trigger your smoking, such as ash trays on nearby tables or certain friends who smoke. You also could be encouraged to get emotional support from your friends and relatives who might be a great help when you eventually decide to quit.

Another often useful technique is called "focused smoking." Basically, it involves rapidly smoking several cigarettes in a row, without stopping. Usually a room with little or no ventilation is preferred so the smoke gets as thick as possible. And, if it's a really good program, they might even show you some rather repulsive things as you do your focused smoking such as pictures of full ashtrays or jars packed with cigarette butts floating in water. As you can guess, the idea is to make you so sick of the smell and taste of the cigarettes that you never want to have another puff.

The next part of the plan could address the physical addiction. One way you can cope with withdrawal symptoms is to get a prescription for a nicotine skinpatch after you quit smoking. This patch is affixed directly to your skin and gradually releases nicotine into your body. What you are doing is getting hooked on the nicotine that's in the skinpatch instead of the nicotine in cigarettes. You should have very few, if any, serious withdrawal symptoms because you can slowly reduce your nicotine intake by gradually wearing patches that release less nicotine.

There are two major advantages to using nicotine skinpatches to help stop smoking. The first is that although you are still addicted to nicotine, wearing the patch will not expose you to the cancer causing chemicals found in cigarettes. The second is that it will give you a chance to get rid of your old habits that triggered your smoking without having to suffer withdrawal symptoms at the same time. In other words, you might learn to teach yourself to avoid cigarettes after meals or during conversation and still not have to worry about feeling jittery.

You may need to work with more than one caregiver to help you stop smoking. In many cases people turn to physicians to prescribe the nicotine patch and to others to help them develop new habits that discourage smoking. It might also be helpful to write or call the American Cancer Society for some of their literature on stop smoking methods. They can be reached by mail at 1599 Clifton Road, N.E., Atlanta Georgia 30329. The telephone number is 404–320–3333.

Physical Intimacy

Sexuality is a big concern to many people who have physical illnesses. One reason for this is that there are countless medical problems and treatments that can interfere with sexual functioning. Many kinds of surgery in the pelvic area, for example, destroy the nerves that lead to the genitals. These surgeries sometimes make normal sexual functioning impossible. Others who have had the penis or vagina removed choose to have reconstructive surgery where new sex organs are made out of skin or mechanical devices. Of course, these new parts often work quite differently than the originals and may cause a long period of emotional and physical adjustment.

Some people with physical problems are afraid to have sex. Heart attack victims, in particular, often worry that intercourse could put too much stress on their heart. Sexual activity, in fact, has been shown to decrease by over half in people who have had heart attacks. Others are concerned about causing a pregnancy at a time when it would be dangerous for them to deliver a child. Many people whose bodies look different because limbs or breasts were removed worry about how attractive they are to their sex partners. And it's not even necessary to have a part of the body mutilated to worry about your appearance. It's easy to see why some people feel less than sexy in the hospital, with their greasy hair flattened down and a urine bag hanging by their side. Some drugs make facial hair grow on women, and breasts enlarge on men. Finally, the stress of being treated for a serious medical problem causes many people to be less interested in sex.

It's common for people with these problems to give up on sex. They can resign themselves to live with physical problems and assume that nothing can be done. Others firmly believe that nobody could ever be attracted to someone who looks "deformed." Finally, some people don't feel comfortable experimenting with ways of getting pleasure that are different from their past habits. All of these attitudes can prevent consumers from learning more about their sexual problems and getting help when it is so badly needed.

Also, some are embarrassed to ask caregivers about sex. If you are concerned about problems find a practitioner you feel comfortable talking with. As with all other health problems, it's very important to keep informed and know what to expect. Many people who have had heart attacks, for example, should have talked to their practitioners more. Some of them have needlessly stopped being sexually active because they were afraid that it could have caused another attack. Actually, many of these people can safely have sex after only a few months of recovery.

You might want to explore different ways of giving and receiving physical pleasure. If intercourse is impossible because of illness, try touching in other ways. Just holding hands or lying next to someone in bed may be enough. If you are concerned about how you look, refer to "Changes in your appearance" in chapter eight. This section was written to help you learn to be comfortable with your body and have more control over others' reactions to it.

There are many caregivers specially trained to help people who have problems with physical intimacy. Ideally, the clinic or hospital in which you are treated will have someone specializing in this area. If not, you may have to find a practitioner yourself who has had experience working with difficulties like yours. Sex therapy may involve five to ten visits to your caregiver's office. If you choose, you can bring your partner. Both of you may be given "homework" to help you increase your sexual enjoyment. In most cases this will be covered by insurance, providing that you work with a well-qualified practitioner and have a good insurance plan.

Hormones are also sometimes used for people with sexual difficulties. Hormone replacement therapy may improve sexual activity, desire, and erections in men who have abnormally low levels of testosterone. Post menopausal women may benefit from estrogen replacement if they have problems with hot flashes, painful orgasm, or bleeding after intercourse. Each of these treatments, however, has risks that should be carefully considered before starting treatment.

Sexuality and Chronic Illness (Schover & Jensen, 1988) is an excellent book that discusses these and other topics relating to the effect of illness on sexuality. Others that may be of interest to people with arthritis or paralysis are *Arthritis: Living and Loving* (Arthritis Foundation, 1982) and *Sexual Options for Paraplegics and Quadriplegics* (Mooney, Cole, & Chilgren, 1975).

Weight Loss

Being overweight has been associated with many problems, including high blood pressure, back problems, and heart disease. It's often a very serious problem for people with health concerns. It may be essential for them to lose weight to recover and lead healthier, happier lives.

Perhaps one of the most difficult obstacles these people have had to face has been keeping their weight off once it was lost. It's very common to lose a lot of weight, only to gain it all slowly back again in a few months. Until about ten years ago, most weight loss experts hadn't designed diet/exercise programs that would help people keep the weight off once it was gone. Nowadays, however, there is much more emphasis on long-term results. To accomplish this, the good weight loss programs often follow their customers for years after the start of their attempts to lose weight. This follow-up may consist of continued coaching in eating right, exercising, and dealing with stress. It is only with such long-term efforts that most people have a reasonable chance of success. Be sure to ask about the long term results before starting any weight loss program. The program should have statistics telling, on average, exactly how much weight people lost and how long they kept it off.

And remember that crash diets are out. Never lose more than one and one-half pounds each week. Whenever you try to lose weight you are most interested in developing habits that will keep the weight off for good. It will do no good to starve yourself and then eat more in a few weeks. If you do want to lose weight, make it a policy not to make any changes in your eating or exercise habits that you aren't willing to keep up for the rest of your life.

There is even some evidence to show that people whose weight goes up and down because of dieting may be making it more difficult for themselves to lose weight in the future. Perhaps, this is because our bodies "think" there is a food shortage when we are dieting. To guard against starvation in the future they make it easier to store up extra energy in the form of body fat. So the ups and downs of many diets may actually make you put on more weight in the long run.

CHAPTER 8

Coping

"I shall ask for brains instead of a heart; for a fool would not know what to do with a heart if he had one."

—Scarecrow

"I shall take the heart...for brains do not make one happy, and happiness is the best thing in the world."

—Tin Woodsman

(The Wonderful Wizard of OZ,

Baum, 1960)

Your Style

People cope with illness in many different ways. While some people deal with their worries by talking to friends, others are much more reserved. Some try to avoid thinking about the same health problems that others prefer to dwell on most of the time. To make matters more complicated, most of us even cope with illness in different ways at different times during our recoveries.

The ways that people cope with being sick or in the hospital are mostly determined by the coping styles that have helped them in the past. If they have had emotional support from others they may have learned to rely on friends and family. They may have found people to be untrustworthy, however, and instead have learned to keep their feelings and concerns to themselves. When you are sick, you may be able to predict pretty accurately how you will cope with your illness. Just think back to how you have dealt with other stress in the past.

People who have never been seriously ill before though may be caught off guard if they have to cope with a sudden illness. One day it might seem strange to them that they want to know everything about their diagnosis, treatment, and prognosis. The next day they might worry about their sudden need to "shut out" the world and not talk to anyone. They might worry that they are "unstable," a concern that could be shared by friends and relatives.

Allan, a man in his early twenties, had a life-threatening kidney disease. This eventually forced him to choose between going on kidney dialysis for the rest of his life or having a kidney transplant. Because kidney dialysis could have greatly interfered with Allan's active lifestyle he chose the transplant. Unfortunately, the day after the transplant he learned that his new kidney had developed the same problem as the one that had been removed. This meant that sometime in the future he would again have to choose between having another transplant or going on dialysis. And, even if he had a second transplant, there was no guarantee that the next kidney wouldn't also eventually have to be replaced.

When Allan first saw a psychologist after his transplant, he was quite upset. He said that he thought about his failed transplant every day and often worried about his future. Since he was planning on having children some day, he was concerned that his health would interfere with his ability to be a good father. He also found that he needed to get quite a bit of emotional support from others at this difficult time in his life. He would often need to talk to his wife about his many fears. What was particularly striking about Allan was his concern about the way he was coping with his illness. He said that he didn't want to think about his health so often or worry about his future. In fact, his relatives also were concerned and told him that he should be coping with his problems "like a man." Understandably, when he felt depressed or anxious he thought he had failed in his attempts to deal with his problems. His purpose for visiting the psychologist was to "fix" himself so he wouldn't be worried about his future.

Allan was making the mistake of believing that his reactions to his health problems were wrong. He expected just to go on with his life as if nothing important had happened to his body. What he needed to do was learn to trust himself and his reactions which were, of course, perfectly normal. Allan was seriously ill and faced the prospect of a lifetime of kidney problems that threatened both his happiness and his life. He had good reason to be scared. Once he realized this he felt much better about how he had handled his illness. Now he didn't believe he was physically and emotionally sick, but rather saw himself as someone who was coping with the stress of illness in the way that worked best for him.

Someone else, who was in the same situation as Allan, might find that a completely different coping style would work better. One common technique is often referred to as "denial." Basically this means that people choose to say to themselves something like

"This really isn't happening" or "Although my caregivers disagree, I will get over this problem." Denial is sometimes a good way to feel better. This is particularly true when people have a physical illness that can't be cured or will result in their death. To face reality might be too painful for them, and it's often much easier for them to cope by simply pretending that the inevitable won't happen. This was demonstrated in an interesting study of people with sickle cell disease (Nadel & Portadin, 1977). This illness is a hereditary blood problem that can cause chronic pain, infection, eye disease, and early death. The authors found that people who coped with their disease using denial had less depression and pain.

How does a person know how they should react to an illness? Are there experts who can visit your home or hospital room and tell you what the best way to cope would be? No. The person with the most expertise on how you should deal with your emotions is you. Trust yourself and listen to what feels right for you.

Trusting your emotional reactions is an important part of taking an active role in your own care. This is because when people don't have confidence in their emotions they often doubt their ability to make rational decisions. They reason,"How could anyone who gets as upset as me ever hope to make good decisions about treatment?" Thus, they might not educate themselves and could turn over the decision making power to others.

But what if your natural emotional style is to deny the reality of your illness or shift all the responsibility for your recovery on to others? Doesn't this mean that it would be stressful to know about and direct your own care? The answer is usually yes. Changing your natural style will be uncomfortable for you. You will be forced to learn things you don't want to know and you will have to make decisions that will be difficult to make. When faced with these problems you need to ask yourself how much emotional comfort you are willing to sacrifice in order to receive higher quality care. Are you willing to be more depressed or frightened in the interests of your recovery? Faced with this question, most people, even those who deny the most, would answer "yes." They realize it's probably worth it to sacrifice some comfort in order to increase the chances of a better recovery.

The people mentioned above with sickle cell disease are a good example of some who have to make a trade-off between the comfort of denial and physical well-being. While denying their physical symptoms may improve their outlook on living, it is also a habit that could easily prevent them from receiving prompt medical care. They may ignore the beginning signs of problems and not report them to their caregiver until they become severe. This may be especially serious when they come down with infections, something to which they are prone throughout their lives (Thomas & Holbrook, 1987). Some professionals even have suggested that people who endanger their own lives by using denial should be considered to have a mental illness (Strauss, Spitzer, & Muskin, 1990).

To restate, your natural style of coping with illness will probably be the most comfortable for you emotionally. It may be easier to deny the seriousness of your situation or to rely on others to make your decisions for you. This doesn't mean there's anything wrong with you or that you are weak. When you are sick, pay attention to your own style and respect it for how it has helped you in the past. At the same time, be aware that if you do tend to be a less than active consumer, you could be endangering your recovery. You need to decide how much of the discomfort of learning about and directing your treatment you can tolerate in the interests of getting higher quality care.

These conflicts will probably not occur in the person whose natural tendency is to get as much information as possible on illness. It would actually be much more stressful for this person not to ask every question he or she could think of or to avoid second guessing each move made by caregivers. Being passive would be threatening by making the person feel out of control. They would fear this sense of powerlessness far more than they would fear knowing too much. It's understandable that this person would be a nightmare for some practitioners. Their sacrifice, if they decide to treat him or her, will be to give up their own total control over care. While they are accustomed to directing of their customers' treatments, they now have to turn much of this control over to the person they are trying to help. The result will be an ongoing bargaining process between caregiver and customer, each trying get more control through the duration of treatment.

Another emotional reaction you might experience is anger. You might be furious at a practitioner for not doing what you want or for making a mistake. You can often use your anger to your advantage though when you are ill. To do this, look at the anger as being the same thing as fear. For example, instead of just being angry at your caregiver for forgetting your appointment, ask yourself what you are afraid will happen because that person didn't show up. It may be that you are afraid you won't have the time to get the treatment you need to recover. In other words, you could think that the broken appointment was your last chance. Another person, though, may be afraid that the missed appointment meant that the caregiver thought there was no chance of recovery. To that person, the broken appointment may be interpreted as a signal that they will never get better.

Obviously these two people, faced with the same situation, need to do totally different things to overcome their fears. The first person will need to do something to make sure he or she gets the needed treatment, perhaps before leaving the hospital or before the caregiver leaves for another city. Remember that this person was afraid of not getting the necessary care. The other person, who was afraid that the missed appointment meant there was no hope of recovery, needs to get accurate information on prognosis. Instead of demanding the proper treatment, this person may need to ask more questions or do more research on his or her illness.

By looking at the causes of anger, different people might do different things to calm their fears and improve the quality of their care. To them the anger actually was helpful. They used it as a signal to look at what they were afraid of in the first place. It was also was a great motivater, pushing them to take appropriate action in their own behalf.

Depending On Others

People differ in their need to rely on others. While some want to turn to friends, relatives, and caregivers to make their decisions for them, others want to do it all themselves. Those who want to control their own treatments may actually feel threatened by depending on others. This is how caregivers often feel when they are hospitalized. Suddenly they have an illness and they may have little power to cure themselves. The same people who have a higher need to control may be the ones who do the most research on their illnesses. They may insist on visiting the best caregiver, even if it means going to a different country. These people can go into a whirlwind of activity in preparation for surgery or other treatment. This could include taking vitamins, having a will written, and doing research on every conceivable form of therapy. This desire to understand and control what happens has helped people save their own lives. It also has changed the course of many treatments, not always in the way caregivers might have preferred.

One man had a particularly difficult time giving up control. He was a very energetic and hard working business leader who had founded a thriving company. Although he and his wife were happy in their marriage he was also in charge of most important decisions related to his family. In short, he was the boss, both at home and at work.

When he was in his 50s he was diagnosed as having a type of cancer that would almost certainly cause his death within a year. Even so, he was offered medication that would probably make his cancer go into remission for much of that time. Once in remission, he would be able to do many of the enjoyable things that he had little time for earlier in his life when he was so preoccupied with business. But at the end of his remission, he would again be faced with uncomfortable cancer treatments that had no guarantee of success.

To the amazement of his family and caregivers, he chose to stop his cancer treatment even though it would have given him a good chance of living comfortably for another year. He realized that without the medicine he would almost certainly die within the next few weeks. In his words:

> *"In my business I was in charge, and I was never a gambling man there. To go on now with my cancer treatment means to gamble with my life, and I may live or*

die even if I do take the medication. I would rather not take that medicine and be certain of my own death, rather than not know if I will survive or not."

This was a good example of what one person was willing to do to stay in charge. It also illustrates the fact that the desire to stay in control is one reason many people don't follow caregivers' advice. So, while the preference to be in charge can help you be a more knowledgeable consumer, it can also change the course of your recovery. In this case, the man's values were different from his caregivers'. His decision to let himself die kept him in control.

A different coping style involves habitually turning to others to make decisions. Quite often people with this style have selected friends or family members to accompany them to the hospital who are quite willing to assume the role of "guard dogs" by looking out for their well being. People with this style are often described as rather dependent people who get emotional support from others. Often it is very comforting to them if they can put themselves in the hands of someone they trust and let them take over their treatment. They are much more likely to talk to others about their problems. It is usually important for them to be close to people throughout an illness and to know that these people will be there for them after they recover.

There is a lot to be said for this coping style. People who use it often have less anxiety and may report much smoother, uneventful recoveries. They tend to ask for help when they need it rather than trying to do everything themselves. The problem with this style of course is that these people may not be as likely to know when they are being given the wrong treatment. And even if they know, they are less likely to be assertive and demand improvements in their care.

Getting Sick And Being Diagnosed

You might be able to have an impact on your care when you first get sick or are just diagnosed. It's at these times that you can often begin to learn more about your problem and to lay the groundwork for your care. Soon after your diagnosis, your library research should certainly be well under way and you may be looking for second and third opinions. One problem is you may be under so much stress that it could be taxing to work in your own behalf. Because of this, you might find you have to do a particularly difficult balancing act between being an informed consumer and respecting the ways you have learned to cope emotionally with illness, which may be by denial or reliance on others.

It might be impossible for you to find a comfortable middle ground between depending on others and actively looking out for your own best interests. And nowhere is this problem likely to be worse than when you first get sick or are newly diagnosed, times when emotions are likely to be strongest and confusion about illness and treatment the greatest. The exception to this, of course, is if you are someone who naturally likes getting lots of information about your illness.

Even if you have learned to rely on others to make your decisions for you though you may find you have skills that will help you get better care. Here, you may be very adept in getting others to help you with your research and find the most competent caregivers. At the same time that you rely on others to do much of the leg work for you, you will need to fight your habit of automatically accepting and trusting the judgment of others over your own.

Let's look at some of the things that could cause you to lose confidence in your ability to make good decisions when you first get sick. It is then that you may have to endure unfamiliar tests and treatments. People might ask you personal or embarrassing questions and perform uncomfortable exams. If you are admitted to the hospital you might be seen in the emergency room or the intensive care unit, each with its own collection of frightening machines. A bright red "crash cart" outside your door, complete with electric paddles for reviving you in case of a heart attack, is an especially menacing piece of equipment for most people. You may have other machines in your room that click, buzz, or pump throughout the night and prevent you from getting much sleep.

Understandably, many people feel frightened and vulnerable at these times. People commonly have panic attacks, especially those who feel most frightened by the prospect of losing control over their bodies. Others report feeling "unreal" and may enter dream-like states when they feel threatened. Some lead themselves to believe that their tests or treatments are being given to someone else. If they are told, for example, that they could die during surgery they might feel as if they were watching their caregiver give someone else that bad news. Finally, some people try to expect the worst will happen. They may either tell themselves that their diagnoses will be serious or their treatments will not work (Register, 1987, p.7.). Their intention is often to prepare themselves for the worst in order to avoid a shock later on.

Many of the ways people cope with illness lower their anxiety. These reactions are especially important early on in treatment, often when people are first diagnosed or admitted to the hospital. The point to remember is that these are probably normal reactions. When they occur don't let them frighten you or make you have less confidence in your ability to make good decisions.

On the other hand, learning your diagnosis might not be a stressful time at all. To some people it is a great relief (Register, 1987). These are often those who have suffered a long time and are relieved to finally learn what's wrong with them. In fact, they might feel elated, even if the illness is serious. At least they know what the problem is and can try to plan for treatment. These people often don't have as many problems in dealing with the emotional shock of being diagnosed. Because of this, they may be more prepared than most to learn about their illnesses.

One problem these people sometimes must contend with is the reactions of others to their relief at being diagnosed. A spouse for example, may wonder why they aren't upset. They may be seen as someone who has trouble "dealing with" illness or as trying to "cover up" their true emotions. The logic usually is that if they aren't upset and "work through" their feelings they will suffer in the long run. There is relatively little scientific evidence to support this belief (Wortman & Silver, 1989). Damage can be done, however, if you doubt your own natural ability to cope with illness and to understand your own care. Again, you should remember to trust yourself and your ability to get high-quality treatment.

Being Treated

As discussed earlier, denial can cause some problems. A good example of such problems often occurs with people who have had head injuries. Because of the physical changes in these peoples brains, many are no longer able to think as clearly as before. Some become confused, tire easily, and have serious problems with memory. Others notice personality changes and have temper outbursts at even minor frustrations.

Such problems are often the most frightening thing these people have ever had to endure. Suddenly they can't remember things they have known for years. It may be impossible for them to carry on normal conversations with friends. It is understandable then that these people use denial. They feel that they can't face their problems. Because of their denial, they often insist that they have not changed much as a result of their head injuries. Even though they can't remember what they had for breakfast, they often go back to work at the same jobs they held before their injury. They also may refuse help from caregivers who might be able to help them improve their memories, become more organized, or control their emotions. Of course when they go back to work without this training they eventually fail. Most are either fired or told to find less demanding positions elsewhere. This is the point where their denial often breaks down. They can no longer pretend that they haven't changed.

When they are no longer able to deny the seriousness of their problems, people with head injuries usually notice a great increase in anxiety. Although it's uncomfortable, it is necessary for them to feel this way before they will accept the help they so desperately need. Anxiety then, is helpful because it motivates them to change. A certain amount of anxiety might also be good for other people who are suffering from illness and need to take a more active role in their own care (Janis, 1958). One of the goals of this book, in fact, is often to make people anxious and, therefore, to motivate people to look out for their own best interests.

Perhaps the times you should put up with more anxiety are the moments when you are really able to have an impact on your own care. Let's consider the example of a person having a heart attack.

When the person first notices chest pain and shortness of breath, it is obviously not the time to use denial. All this will do is delay the trip to the emergency room where the person could receive life-saving care. This is the time to put up with anxiety and admit that one's life is in danger. Once admitted to the hospital and given proper care, the person may be able to have much less impact her treatment. This is the time that a little denial might help the person feel better emotionally. It also gives time to charge the person's emotional batteries for the long and difficult recovery ahead, a time when the person will need to be a far more active participant in researching and planning treatment. Upon discharge from the hospital, denial might again work against the person because it could discourage the person from exercising properly, eating a healthy diet, and going to the hospital again in the event of more problems.

You may wish to keep this in mind if you decide to use any of the pain or anxiety management strategies described in chapter six. Some are best suited for people who are going through a period in which denial or distraction would be useful. Imagery techniques in particular are often the best route for people who can't have much of an impact on their own care anyway and need to lose themselves in thought. You may decide to use other strategies at times when you should pay attention to your physical symptoms. Muscle relaxation techniques (Miller, Leinbach, and Brody, 1989) and diaphragmatic breathing are well suited for this because they help you to pay attention to different body sensations that may signal important changes in your condition.

Some people find that it is helpful to have a single room in the hospital. This makes it easier for a person to practice relaxation strategies, sleep through the night, and visit privately with friends and relatives. If you want a private room, be sure to ask for one to be reserved well ahead of time. And surprisingly, it usually only costs a few dollars a day to buy yourself this privacy. Remember also that rooms with windows are the best. If you are really lucky (or assertive), you might even get a window that actually opens. Some research (Ulrich, 1983) has shown that people who have pleasant views from their hospital windows feel better faster and need less medicine to control pain.

Before you go into the hospital, also be sure to pack things that will make you feel at home. These might include your robe, pajamas, and list of telephone numbers. Some people bring inexpensive pictures for the wall along with adhesive-backed hooks to hang them up. Don't forget your radio, tape recorder, or compact disc player. Other ideas include books, photo albums, and even small refrigerators stocked with favorite foods.

Try to avoid being admitted to the hospital on a weekend (Boardroom, 1991) or during a holiday. The primary caregivers are usually home or on vacation at these times so your treatment might just be postponed until they return anyway.

Leaving The Hospital

To a sick person, a hospital can be a very comforting place. There are often many highly skilled caregivers there who use sophisticated medical equipment to help people survive life-threatening emergencies. Help is never more than minutes away. It's understandable then that after people are sent home from the hospital they often feel frightened and vulnerable when this care is no longer available. One common reaction at this time is for people to rely more on family and friends for both emotional support and help with physical problems. As in earlier stages of diagnosis and treatment, one danger is that people may rely too much on others and not actively try to understand their own care.

This is a serious problem when people don't get the treatment they need once they leave the hospital. Poor care after leaving the hospital may be especially common now that health insurance plans are doing so much to spend less money. Needed services, such as home visits by nurses, medical equipment to be used in the home, or counseling may be denied in order to keep costs down. The caregivers themselves may also drop the ball. They can be working so hard helping people in the hospital that they neglect the needs of their customers once they go home. For each of these reasons, then, it's very important to continue being an informed and assertive consumer even after you leave the hospital.

To do this, begin planning for your trip home long before it occurs. Talk to your caregivers about the different kinds of treatment or help you will need when you leave the hospital. For example, have you thought about how you will go to the pharmacy to get your medication? Will you be able to bathe yourself and prepare the kinds of foods you should eat? Who will be nearby to help if you suddenly have a medical emergency? These are the types of things you should prepare for well in advance. It may be particularly important to get your insurance company to approve payment for these and other services ahead of time to avoid uncomfortable or even dangerous delays.

If you are in the hospital it should have a social service agency to help arrange for your care once you leave. For example, you may meet with a social worker, someone from Hospice (if you are terminally ill), a nurse, and so forth before you are scheduled to go home. It is this person's duty to see that you get the needed treatment after you are discharged. If you aren't satisfied with the discharge plans they have arranged for you, you might threaten to refuse to leave the hospital (Boardroom, 1991). Many hospitals are under so much pressure to discharge people early (and thereby cut costs) that your refusal may get them to arrange the care that you need.

Also be certain to take enough medication and other supplies home with you from the hospital to last a long time. It's surprising how many people are sent home without enough pills to keep them comfortable for more than a few days. Another advantage to going home with plenty of supplies is that your insurance plan may pay more for these things if they are given to you while you are hospitalized. If you have to go to the pharmacy or drug store on your own you might be forced to pay the whole bill yourself.

Of course, be sure you know what your medications are prescribed for and how to use them properly. Some hospital administrators (Orr, 1990) have stated that as many as 40% of the people who have gone back into the hospital were re-admitted because they didn't take their medication correctly.

When many people leave the hospital they are disappointed about their recovery. Either their treatment didn't work as they had hoped or unexpected problems happened. Looking back, it may be clear that they just didn't get good care. When this happens, it may cause special problems for more active and knowledgeable consumers. It is these people who are most likely to blame themselves for what went wrong. They may tell themselves things like "I should have known not to go to that hospital" or "If I had studied just a little more I would not have gone to that caregiver."

This harsh self-criticism is a strategy many people use to control their own behavior. They think that by punishing themselves they will learn to make better choices about health care. This approach usually doesn't work. Instead of motivating people to do better next time, it usually causes them to have less confidence in their ability to make good decisions.

Clearly, this strategy can have a very corrosive effect on one's self-confidence. It also may result in people taking a less, rather than more, active role in understanding their own care. Since this is the opposite of what you want to do, it's probably better just to accept the fact that you will make mistakes. This will mean trying to learn from past mistakes so you will be able to make better decisions about health care in the future.

Once you go home you might be interested in meeting others with your illness. There are many support and self-help groups these days and you just might be able to find one that would help you get in touch with some of these people. Each group is usually composed of people that all have a specific medical and/or psychological problem. If you look through a newspaper there is a good chance you will find a section devoted entirely to announcing the meetings of groups. You could also contact the National Self-Help Clearinghouse at 22 West 43rd Street, Room 620, New York, N.Y. 10036 [telephone 212–642–2944] for free help locating the right group. When you find one, you might notice meetings ranging from Alcoholics Anonymous to Survivors of Cancer. People often attend these meetings to learn about how other people have coped with illness or have received better health care. Often spouses are welcome to attend but you should probably call and inquire first, since many groups place a high priority on confidentiality.

If there isn't a group to fit your needs, consider forming one of your own. Take advantage of the free advertising often provided by newspapers to announce your meeting. You might also contact your caregivers to see if they have any customers who might be interested in attending.

Many people need help carrying out their usual activities after they leave the hospital. It may be more difficult for them to mow the lawn, chauffeur the kids to and from piano lessons, and buy groceries. Out of necessity then, they need to ask for help from others when these responsibilities become too great. Often it's very helpful for them to keep lists of people who can help (Register, 1987). They might have one list of baby sitters, one of people who would be willing to run to the store, and another listing those who could pick up their children from school if they can't go themselves.

Changes In Your Appearance

One of the most difficult problems many ill people have to deal with is a change in their physical appearance. Not only can this profoundly affect their self-esteem but it can easily change the way others treat them. Unfortunately, if you don't "look right" you may be invited to fewer social events, people may ask rude questions, and others might be less friendly. There are many changes that can occur as a result of illness. Some people have arms or legs amputated. Women have mastectomies and there are many head and facial surgeries that can leave people deformed. Sometimes medications cause baldness or swollen faces.

What's particularly troubling about changes in physical appearance is the fact that you probably had no choice about whether or not the changes would occur. Most likely you needed to have the surgery or medication that caused the change, possibly to save your life. You also had no choice about having the illness in the first place. Your problem was certainly nothing you asked for and most likely there was nothing you could have done to prevent it. You also may have little or no control over the stares of others. When you are in public many people, not just children, look at your scar or missing limb or whatever it is that makes you different. Understandably, these problems leave many feeling out of control.

There are, however, a number of things that you can do that might help you regain some control. These are designed to put you back in charge of both your medical treatment and your self-esteem. One strategy is to train others about what to say or do about your appearance (Rice, 1989). As an example, imagine that you had a facial deformity caused by surgery. One of the most difficult moments for you then might be when relatives want to take family pictures. While some people feel very comfortable having themselves photographed, it might be an experience that others dread. If it's something you don't want to have done, tell people. Say something simple like "since my surgery I just haven't felt comfortable having my picture taken." If they argue with you (and they probably will) don't give in. Remember that you are in charge and it's how you feel that counts, regardless of the reassurances of others.

In some cases you will need to educate people about what the changes in your body do and do not mean. Some may think that because your face looks different you are mentally retarded. Rather than being insulted and feeling depressed, try taking charge. You could tell them that just because you look different you still are as smart as you were before. Another person with a facial deformity may want to tell her husband whether or not she wants to be touched on the face. Others might take charge like this because of changes such as the removal of a breast or limb.

People also want to take charge when they feel embarrassed in public. Some choose to do this by making eye contact with starers. This will this usually make the other people look away and increase your feelings of control over their rudeness. I remember hearing of one married couple with dwarfism who took this a step farther. Whenever they would go out in public people would stare and point. They eventually played a rather mischievous game and started pointing back. This always put a quick end to the inconsiderate behavior.

When you are in public also remember that people looked at you before the change in your appearance occurred. All glances and stares are not because of your "defect" but may be just a natural result of being in a public place. Just because someone looks at you doesn't mean they think you are different. So be careful that you aren't oversensitive, thinking that every time others look at you it's because they are critical of how you look. In fact, you may want to pay special attention to the many positive responses you get from others. Try to remember each time someone says something nice about your appearance or admires something you are wearing.

It may be especially helpful to decide how important the opinions of others are to you. If they don't like you or are critical of your appearance does it make that much difference to you? Although it certainly won't be pleasant, is their opinion of you enough to make you feel so bad about yourself?

Sometimes people who have had major changes in their appearance will avoid thinking about their bodies. These people also can try not to talk about it, and may even bathe less often. Along with this may be a tendency to avoid things that used to give them physical pleasure, since these things would force them to think about how their body looks or feels. It is very important for many people to "reconnect" with their bodies and experience the things that used to give them physical pleasure (Rice, 1989). There are many ways this can be done. Perhaps you used to enjoy taking long showers. You might decide to get into the habit of spending more time in the shower and learn again to enjoy the feeling of the hot water on your body. You might be interested in starting an exercise program. When people exercise they have to pay attention to how their bodies feel before, during, and after their workouts. Not only may this help you reconnect, but it could help you regain the confidence and pride you once had in yourself. People have found many other solutions ranging from chocolate to sex. Some people buy new clothes. Do whatever helps.

You may find that it's especially difficult to think about your appearance just after it has changed. If this happens, don't force yourself to do anything that's too uncomfortable. Instead, gradually try to pay more attention to the part of you that is different. If you had a facial scar you might glance at it once or twice a day for a month. After that you might want to look at it for a longer time or to feel it. Not only may this help you become more comfortable with yourself, but it could help you notice gradual improvement. This is especially important to people who tend to see their disfigurements as "all or nothing." In other words, they see themselves as either having a terrible scar or no scar at all. There is no middle ground. Noticing gradual changes could help them realize that they are slowly healing and looking more "normal" all the time. It will be up to them to try to be satisfied with gradual improvement and not expect 100% recovery in just a short while.

Depression

Depression is a problem familiar to many people who are coping with illness. It is especially likely to strike those who think they have no control over their lives. In other words, people who can't make choices about their care or think that their illnesses won't get better are most likely to be depressed.

There are many symptoms of depression. Perhaps most often, people who are depressed feel a sense of hopelessness and helplessness. They think that there is nothing they can do to feel better. Some people notice that their sleep changes. Often they find themselves waking up early in the morning and not being able to fall back to sleep, even though they are tired. Sometimes appetites change. While some depressed people notice that they eat more, others lose the desire to eat much at all. Many people complain that they have trouble making decisions. Choices as simple as what to have for dinner may be more than they can handle. People who are depressed sometimes have difficulty starting projects and notice that they don't have nearly as much energy as they have had in the past. Other symptoms include crying spells, lowered sex drive, less enjoyment of things, and even thoughts of suicide.

It's important not to confuse some of these symptoms with normal thoughts and behavior often seen in people being treated for medical problems. Many people recovering from surgery certainly don't have much energy, appetite, sex drive, or ambition — not because of depression, but because they are sick. It's only when these symptoms are worse than would be expected from the physical problems alone that depression is suspected.

There is a myth that it is always healthy for people who have suffered major losses to be depressed (Wortman & Silver, 1989). The reasoning is that everyone needs to "confront" or "work through" problems at some time or another. If this isn't done just after the loss occurred, many people believe that it will eventually happen in the future and may be much worse. Some people who have been paralyzed for example, are often encouraged to talk about their feelings soon after their injury. Many caregivers do this with the best of intentions, thinking it will save the person from having to deal with more serious depression later on.

Although this does help many people, it is not for everyone. This is because some people don't feel depressed, even after suffering major traumas such as the death of a spouse (Clayton, Halikas, & Maurice, 1971) or a serious injury (Lawson, 1976). Again, your decision whether or not to talk about your problems will depend on your own feelings. You may want to confide in others. You may also be one of those people though who just doesn't need to talk. It may be that you aren't feeling that bad in the first place. It may also not be your "style" to confide in others, something that could just make you feel more uncomfortable. Finally, you might be trying not to think about your problems, a sometimes comforting technique referred to earlier as denial.

The point is that the way you choose to get over your depression will be unique. When others encourage you to get better a certain way, they may not realize that their way is not necessarily the best thing for you. Instead, it's better for you to have the confidence in yourself to make your own decisions about how to feel better. If you decide you need to talk, then talk. If you think it would be better to keep quiet, then don't say a word. And, if you feel fine to begin with, don't doubt your own common sense by listening to those who insist you are ignoring your problem by not feeling depressed.

Many people feel less depressed when they learn to be more involved in their own care. When they understand their illnesses and know how to help themselves, even just a little, at least they feel they have some power. This is often one key to recovery. Other people, though, are just the opposite. When they start to be informed consumers they may feel more depressed.

Earlier in this book anxiety was described as a side effect of learning to be a more active consumer. It's just one more thing that you must suffer in order to receive better care. For some, it is the same with depression. They have to put up with more depression when they become better consumers. It's often discouraging to know about all the things that could go wrong. It's difficult to take on more responsibility for yourself at a time when you are so sick. But again, there is a tradeoff. It may be up to you to decide how much more depression you are willing to tolerate in order to be a more involved consumer.

Below are a few ideas to help you with your own depression. Keep in mind that not all of these things work for everyone because we all have different styles.

1. Try forcing yourself to do something fun, even if you don't feel like it. Don't let your lack of enthusiasm keep you from trying something fun. You may be surprised how quickly you come out of your rut when you do something enjoyable.
2. Try making friends with someone else in the hospital. You may want to complain about the food or even just compare scars. But the conversation might give both of you a lift.
3. Ask for antidepressant medication to help you with your mood. Sometimes this helps quite a bit in a short time.
4. Try taking more control over your treatment. To do this you may need to study more, ask more questions, learn pain or anxiety management skills, or be more assertive.
5. Ask yourself if you have a habit of being too hard on yourself. Pay attention to the way you talk about yourself. Do you say things like "If only I wasn't so..." or "It's bad that I don't have the courage to...." If so, you may be in the habit of being far too critical of your own abilities. It's understandable that this can contribute to depression. Instead, try to say more permissive and accepting things in place of the put-downs that usually go through your mind.

You might want to try something like "Even though I have this problem, I still am worthwhile." You may also want to purchase the enjoyable book *Talking to Yourself* (Butler, 1981). It is written, in part, to help you lift your depression by changing the way you think.

6. Make yourself laugh. Tell a joke, watch a silly movie, or play a trick on someone.
7. Ask yourself if you are being realistic about your worries. Many people have a tendency to "catastrophize," and think the worst will happen. Try to spot those concerns about things that have little chance of actually occurring.
8. Try to spend more time with friends and relatives. Do something to make a visit to you more enjoyable. Ask that board games or cards be brought to your room so your relatives' children will have something to play with when they are there. Tell people to visit at mealtime so you can all order a pizza as you would if you were home. At the same time, try not to get more depressed if some of your friends don't visit. Remember, some of them might be frightened to come to see you. Others may wait for an invitation. Without it they will stay away out of respect for your privacy.
9. Spend two hours every day pampering yourself. Just think of the hedonistic pleasures you have been missing. Now that you are sick nobody will ever think you are being frivolous for paying to have your feet or back massaged or for buying the biggest box of chocolates in town. Make your two hours your time to do whatever you like.
10. Remember that you may need to arrange for extra emotional support from others in the evenings or at night. When people are tired and worn down late in the day they are naturally going to have a more difficult time emotionally. This is also the time of day that many visitors go home. You may need to make a special request if you need some company to help lift your spirits at later hours.
11. Talk to clergy. Many people find comfort speaking with others about spirituality. Clergy are usually able to come

to your hospital room in accordance with your needs.

12. Don't compare your recovery to those of people who have recovered faster than you. Remember, some people need more time to get better. Expecting yourself to keep pace with the person down the hall is inviting disappointment.

Because of an illness or injury, people often aren't able to do something they once enjoyed. Perhaps they have to be less physically active and can't go back to work. Or maybe they have to take medications that make it difficult for them to think clearly or drive a car. Often people don't become discouraged about these things until after they leave the hospital. In part, this is because when they are in the hospital they are still in a period of denial. During this time, although they are told that they won't be able to do certain things, it really doesn't affect them until they try to do something and fail. It is at this point that they have to face reality. One consequence of this reality is often depression.

But stop and think for a minute what this depression can mean. It often means that you are trying to have control over your world. You may be looking for ways to do things with your family or be more productive at work. You could be learning how to get around the city again, this time using public transportation. You may even be looking for new hobbies that you can enjoy. All these things can be very healthy and satisfying in the long run. Before you master them though, you could feel very frustrated and depressed. So when you feel down, keep in mind that it may be a signal that you are going through a very difficult, but productive, period in your life. Your depression could mean that you are trying to be active and in control of yourself again.

Taking Control

One of this book's main goals has been to help readers develop a sense of control over their own health care. Recently scientists have learned about the importance feelings of control may have for both our mental and physical health. Some of the first research in this area was done with animals, which were exposed to stress that they had no power to control. For example, some were given mild electric shocks from which they could not escape (Seligman & Maier, 1967; Visintainer & Seligman, 1983). No matter what they did they would still occasionally feel the electric current through the floors or walls of their cages. After a short time many of these animals usually laid down and seemed to give up trying to get away from the shocks. Later on, when they were given the chance to escape the shocks by going to another part of their cages, the animals didn't move. In other words, they learned to be helpless.

Just like the animals in the earlier experiments, people being treated for health problems may learn to be helpless. The original cause of this may be the development of their illness in the first place. They probably could not have prevented their illness and certainly never asked for it to happen. Or, they may have had a caregiver who kept them in the dark about their disease. This caregiver may also have "taken over" by prescribing treatments without their knowledge. Family members may have entered into the picture, making decisions even if the ill person wanted to make different choices. Finally, the treatment itself may have robbed the person of control. Medication may have interfered with the ability to think clearly or surgery could have made it impossible to get out of bed.

It's not surprising that many people, just like the animals given unavoidable shock, soon feel powerless. This sense of helplessness may stop them from directing their own treatments confidently by learning about their problems and trying to get better care when it is needed. Both the caged animals and the people in the hospital have had much of their power taken away. As a result, both may sit and suffer rather than try to help themselves.

Helplessness may do more harm to people than just make them poor consumers of health care. More and more scientific studies are suggesting that both animals and humans may be more likely to suffer from disease if they have learned to be helpless. In one study (Visintainer & Seligman, 1983) researchers injected live cancer cells in rats. One of the groups was occasionally given mild electric shocks. The second group was given the same shocks but was able stop them by pressing a lever. In other words, this second group was given control over the electricity.

It is striking that only 27% of the animals that could not control the shocks survived, while 63% of the rats that had been able to turn off the electricity had no signs of cancer at all. The rats that were helpless died more than twice as often as those that had learned to control the shocks. The authors concluded that being helpless increased the chances that the animals would die of cancer.

Of course, it would be a mistake to make any conclusions about humans from studies done on rats. However, a few experiments have been done to discover a link between people's feelings of helplessness and their physical and emotional well being. Some studies, for example, have shown that people who feel helpless visit physicians more often, die earlier, and are more likely to have infectious diseases (Peterson & Seligman, 1987). Another (Langer, Janis, & Wolfer 1975) showed that hospitalized people who felt that they had more control over stress asked for fewer sedatives and pain killers. They were also judged by nurses to have less anxiety.

One very interesting study (Langer & Rodin, 1976) looked at what happened when elderly nursing home residents were given more control over their lives. Before the study, this was a group of people who had almost all of their decisions made for them. They didn't have to worry about what to prepare for meals, what to wear, or even to remember to take medication on time. They really had no responsibility for doing much of anything.

The authors of the study decided to make some changes in the lives of some of the residents. One day a group of them were called together for a meeting. Among other things they were told that they were responsible for arranging their own furniture, deciding when they wanted to visit their friends, and making choices about what they wanted to do for entertainment. They were also encouraged to make any complaints or suggestions about the facility known to staff members. Finally, a box of potted plants was passed to each of the residents. They were told that, if they wanted, they could select a plant for themselves. They were also informed that if they decided to have a plant they would be responsible for taking care of it.

Three weeks later, these residents were compared to those who didn't have the opportunity to take care of a plant and were not reminded that they could make many decisions for themselves. Almost three-fourths of those who did not receive a plant became more debilitated, even in that short period of time. They were less alert and active, not as happy, and did fewer things socially than those who were encouraged to make decisions for themselves. In contrast, 93% of those who were reminded that they could have more control showed improvement in these same areas. As long as a year and a half later the people who were helped to have more power still had better moods and were more active. What was particularly striking at this time though was that these people died only half as often as those who were not encouraged to take responsibility for themselves (Rodin & Langer, 1977).

Nobody knows for sure why animals and people seem to feel better and possibly live longer if they think they have some control over what happens to them. Scientists have guessed that feeling helpless somehow makes it more difficult for the immune system to do its job. A weakened immune system could cause all sorts of problems, including infections and an increased risk of cancer. Anyway it will probably be many years before we know for certain just how this process works. In the meantime, we can still make use of the knowledge that helplessness probably makes it more likely that we will get sick.

It is the most skilled and sensitive caregivers who try to nurture whatever sense of power and control already lives in their customers. These are the ones who encourage ill people to make their own decisions, even about things that may seem trivial. When they walk out of the hospital room of someone confined to bed they may ask "Do you want your door left open or closed?" While this might seem unimportant, it may give the sick person another way to have some control over the world. If the door is closed, they will probably have more privacy and a quieter room. If left open, they may have the chance to talk with people who happen to walk by in the hallway. Such an "unimportant" matter actually may greatly change this person's world. And if the person had not been asked what they wanted, they may have had a difficult time finding someone who would have opened or closed the door for them later on.

Of course, it's probably even more important for ill people to feel a sense of control over crucial decisions about their own health care. Leaving the door open or closed will help, but only if they also feel the sense of security that often comes from being in charge.

If you're looking for some ideas about how to feel more in control in the hospital read through the following list. I hope it will get you thinking and help you come up with some more ideas of your own.

1. Try learning some anxiety or pain control techniques. These are described in detail in chapter six and are often an important part of people's emotional and physical recovery.
2. Ask for a second opinion. This may be especially important if you are concerned that you are not getting the proper treatment.
3. Ask to be taken to a place where they normally do not take customers. Wouldn't you like to go down to the hospital cafeteria where the visitors eat? How about asking to be taken across the street to that Italian restaurant you see out your window? Your hospital should have already have a system worked out for giving customers "day passes" to allow these kinds of excursions.
4. Look at your problem as a more of a challenge rather than as a threat (Folkman, 1984). Just seeing your illness as a threat is only likely to make you scared.
5. Tell a caregiver or a friend that the timing of their visit isn't convenient for you and that you would like them to return in five minutes. This is more symbolic than anything else but can mean a great deal to people whose caregivers barge in and out of their rooms at all hours of the day.
6. Strike an agreement that your lab tests will be performed only once a day. One person (Cousins, 1979, pp. 28-29.) had blood drawn and stored in a bottle once every three

days of his hospitalization. This way all of the people who needed blood simply drew their samples from this container that was conveniently stored outside his room.

7. Ask at least five questions every day.
8. Become an expert at using all of those little buttons near the side of your bed. Those buttons often change the position of your bed, control the T.V. and radio, and can be used to call the nurses down the hall. Surprisingly, many people never learn to feel comfortable using these controls. Because of this they often wait for others to do many of these simple things for them.
9. Ask that your roommate sleep on his or her side to eliminate nighttime snoring. Sleep is very important to you, especially at a time when you are trying to recover.
10. Set new personal goals. Perhaps your illness has made it impossible for you to achieve some things that you used to value or enjoy. For example, a serious foot injury may make it impossible for you to continue participating in running marathons. Rather than continuing to try to be a competitive runner, try to set your sights on something else. Maybe you need to be satisfied with an occasional jog. Perhaps it is also wise to change your sport to swimming or something else that doesn't hurt your foot. Once your goals have become more realistic, and you see some progress, it may be possible for you to feel as if you have control over your life again (Folkman, 1984).

If the research on the benefits of being in control is right, it makes sense that you might do better physically and emotionally if you learn to call your own shots about health care. This is the point of learning to be a better consumer. Like the people in nursing homes who felt better after watering their own plants, you also might recover faster by being informed and helping to control your own destiny.

References

Aaron, H., & Schwartz, W. B. (1990, January 26). "Rationing Health Care: The Choice Before Us." *Science*. 247, 418-422.

Adler, T. (1989). "Happiness-Health Link Remains Questionable." APA Monitor. January, 9.

Alberti, R. E, & Emmons, M. L. (1988). *Your Perfect Right*. San Luis Obispo, California: Impact Publishers.

Allen, Woody. (1979). *Manhattan*, Woody Allen, screenplay; Rollins-Joffe Productions; Distributed by United Artists.

American Osteopathic Association. (Undated). *Osteopathic Medicine: A Distinctive Branch of Mainstream Medical Care*. Available from AOA, 142 East Ontario Street, Chicago, IL 60611

American Osteopathic Association. (Undated). *An Introduction to Osteopathic Medicine*. Available from AOA, 142 Ontario Street, Chicago IL 60611.

Ammer, C. (1982). *The Common Sense Guide to Mental Health Care*. Brattleboro, VT: Viking-Penguin.

Anderson, E. A. (1987). "Preoperative Preparation For Cardiac Surgery Facilitates Recovery, Reduces Psychological Distress, and Reduces The Incidence of Acute Postoperative Hypertension." *Journal of Consulting and Clinical Psychology*. 55 (4), 513-520.

Arluke, A., Kennedy, L. & Kessler, R. C. (1979) "Reexamining the Sick Role Concept: an Empirical Assessment." *Journal of Health and Social Behavior*, 20, 30-36.

Arthritis Foundation (1982). *Arthritis: Living and Loving: Information About Sex*. (9190, 9197-9182). Atlanta, GA: Arthritis Foundation.

Baum, L. F. (1960). *The Wonderful Wizard of OZ*. (p. 61), New

York, N.Y.: Dover.

Beck, M., Yoffe, E., Carroll, G., Hager, M., Rosenberg, D., & Beachy, L. (1990, December 10). "The Politics of Breast Cancer." *Newsweek*, pp. 62-65.

Beers, M. H., Munekata, M., & Storrie, M. (1990). "The Accuracy of Medication Histories in the Hospital Medical Records of Elderly Persons." *Journal of the American Geriatrics Society*. 38, 1183-1187.

Bergin, A. E., & Lambert, M. J. (1978). "The Evaluation of Therapeutic Outcomes." In S. L. Garfield & A. E. Bergin (Eds.). *Handbook of Psychotherapy and Behavior Change: An Empirical Analysis*. (2nd ed.) (pp. 139-189). New York: John Wiley & Sons.

Berman, H, & Rose, L. (1990). *Choosing the Right Health Care Plan. Consumer Reports* Books.

Blair, S. N., Piserchia, P. V., Wilbur, C. S., & Crowder, J. H. (1986). "A Public Health Intervention Model for Work-Site Health Promotion." *The Journal of the American Medical Association*. 255 (February), 921-926

Bly, J. L., Jones, R. C., & Richardson, J. E. (1986). "Impact of Worksite Health Promotion on Health Care Costs And Utilization." *The Journal of the American Medical Association*. 256 (December), 3235-3240.

Boardroom. (1991). *The Book of Inside Information*. New York, N.Y.: Boardroom Reports, Inc.

Bruno, F. J. (1989). *The Family Mental Health Encyclopedia*. New York, N.Y.: Wiley.

Butler, P. E. (1983). *Talking to Yourself*. San Francisco, California: Harper & Row.

Butler, P. E. (1981). *Self-Assertion for Women*. San Francisco, California: Harper & Row. Staff. (1989, June). Beyond medicare. *Consumer Reports*. pp. 375-386.

Cassileth, B. R. (1989). *The Social Implications of Questionable Cancer Therapies*. Cancer. 63, 1247-1250.

Cassileth, B. R. (1980). "Informed Consent - Why are its Goals Imperfectly Realized?" *New England Journal of Medicine*. 302 (16), 866-900.

Chambless, D. L. & Gracely, E. J. (1989). "Fear of Fear and the Anxiety Disorders." *Cognitive Therapy and Research* 19, pp. 85-88.

Clark, D. M. (1986). "A Cognitive Approach to Panic." *Behavior Research and Therapy*. 24 (4), 461-470.

Clayton, P. J., Halikas, J. A., & Maurice, W. L. (1972). "The Depression of Widowhood." *British Journal of Psychiatry*. 120, 71-78.

Coe, R. M., Prendergast, C. & Psathas, G. (1984). "Strategies for Obtaining Compliance with Medical Regimens." *Journal of the American Geriatrics Society*. 32, 589-593.

Cousins, N. (1979). *Anatomy of an Illness, as Perceived by the Patient*. New York, N. Y.: W. W. Norton & Company, Inc.

Cousins, N. (1983). *The Healing Heart*. New York, N. Y.: W.W. Norton & Company, Inc.

"Crisis in Health Insurance" (1990, August). *Consumer Reports*. pp. 533-549.

Devine, E. C. & Cook, T. E. (1983). "A Meta-Analytic Analysis Of Effects Of Psychoeducational Interventions On Length Of Postsurgical Hospital Stay." *Nursing Research*. 32 (5), 267-274.

Devine, E. C. & Cook, T. E. (1986). "Clinical and Cost-Saving Effects of Psychoeducational Interventions With Surgical Patients: A Meta-Analysis." *Research in Nursing & Health* 9, 89-105.

Eastaugh, S. R. (1986). "Hospital Quality Scorecards, Patient Severity, and the Emerging Value Shopper." *Hospital & Health Services Administration*. November/December, 85-102.

Eisenhauer, E. D., Derveloy, R. J., & Hastings, P. R. (1982). "Prospective Evaluation of Central Venous Pressure (CVP) Catheters in a Large City-County Hospital." *Annals of Surgery*. 196, 560-564.

Ellwood, P. M. (1982). "The American Way of Medical Care 1980-1990." In J. Gay and B. S. Jacobs (Eds.). *Competition in the Marketplace: Health Care in the 1980s* (pp. 77-83). Jamaica, NY: Spectrum Publications.

Felson, B. (1987). "Coronary Artery Disease and Coronary Artery Bypass Graft." In H. Mandell & H. Spiro (Eds.), *When Doctors Get Sick* (pp. 19-27). New York and London: Plenum. [fictitious name]

Findlay, S. (1990). "Deciphering Your Hospital Bill." *U.S. News & World Report*. April 30, 60.

Flood, A. B., Scott, W., R., & Ewy, W. (1984). "Does Practice Make Perfect?" *Medical Care*. 22 (2), 98-114.

Folkman, S. (1984). "Personal Control and Stress and Coping Processes: A Theoretical Analysis." *Journal of Personality and Social Psychology*. 46 (4), 839-852.

Friedman, M. & Ulmer, D. (1984). *Treating Type A Behavior and Your Heart*. New York, N.Y.: Fawcett Crest.

Goldfried, M. R., & Davison, G. G. (1976). *Clinical Behavior Therapy*. New York: Holt, Rinehart, and Winston.

Goldstein, A. & Stainback, B. (1987). *Overcoming Agoraphobia*. New York, N.Y.: Viking Penguin, Inc.

Greenfield, S., Kaplan, S., & Ware, J. E. (1985). "Expanding Patient Involvement In Care." *Annals of Internal Medicine*. 102 (4), 520-528.

Greenfield, S., Kaplan, S., Ware, J. E., & Yano, E. M. (1988). "Patients' Participation in Medical Care: Effects on Blood Sugar Control and Quality of Life in Diabetes." *Journal of General Internal Medicine*. 3, 448-457.

Greenland, P., Mushlin, A. I., & Griner, P. F. "Discrepancies Between Knowledge and Use of Diagnostic Studies In Asymptomatic Patients." *Journal of Medical Education*. 54, 863-869.

Greiner, L., & Weiler, C. (1983). "Early-Stage Breast Cancer: What do Women Know About Treatment Choices? *American Journal of Nursing* 83 (11), 1570.

Griffith, H. W. (1989). *Instructions for Patients*. Lea & Febiger.

Griffith, H. W. (1989). *Complete Guide To Symptoms, Illness & Surgery*. Tucson, AZ: The Body Press.

Hadley, J., Steinberg, E. P., & Feder, J. (1991). "Comparison of Uninsured and Privately Insured Hospital Patients." *Journal of the American Medical Association*. 265 (3), 374-379.

Hamburger, T. (1989, March 8). "State Health Care System is Missing Black Moms." *Minneapolis Star Tribune*

Hartz, A. J., Krakauer, H., Kuhn, E. M., Young, M., Jacobsen, S. J., Greer, G., Muenz, L., Katzoff, M., Bailey, R. C., & Rimm, A. A. (1989). "Hospital Characteristics and Mortality Rates." *The New England Journal of Medicine*. Dec., pp. 1720-1725.

Haug, M. & Lavin, B. (1983) *Consumerism in Medicine: Challenging Physician Authority*. Beverly Hills, CA: Sage.

Hayes-Bautista, D. (1976). "Termination of the Patient-Practitioner Relationship: Divorce, Patient Style." *Journal of Health and Social Behavior*. 17, 12-22.

Hassenfeld, I., & Drew, B. (1989, February). *Men and Women React Differently to Life-Threatening Illnesses*. Notes. Printed by the Acoustic Neuroma Association, P.O. Box 398, Carlisle, PA. 17013.

Hauri, P. (1982). *The Sleep Disorders*. Kalamazoo, Michigan: The Upjohn Company.

Hillman, A. L., Pauly, M. V., & Kerstein, J. J. (1989). "How Do Financial Incentives Affect Physicians' Clinical Decisions and the Financial Performance of Health Maintenance Organizations?" *The New England Journal of Medicine*. 321 (2), 86-92.

Hillman, B. J., Joseph, C. A., Mabry, M. R., Sunshine, J. H., Kennedy, S. D., & Noether, M. (1990, December 6). "Frequency and Costs of Diagnostic Imaging in Office Practice - A Comparison of Self-Referring and Radiologist-Referring Physicians." *The New England Journal of Medicine*. 323 (3), 1604-1608.

Jacobson, E. (1929) *Progressive Relaxation*. Chicago: University of Chicago Press.

Janis, I. L. (1958). *Psychological Stress: Psychoanalytic and Behavioral Studies of Surgical Patients*. New York: Wiley.

Kaplan, S. H., Greenfield, S., & Ware, J. E. (1989). "Assessing the Effects of Physician-Patient Interactions on the Outcomes of Chronic Diseases." *Medical Care*. 27 (3 supplement), S110-S126.

Koek, K., Martin, S. B., & Novallo, A. (Eds.). (1993). *Encyclope-*

dia of Associations. (24th Edition). Detroit, MI: Gale Research, Inc.

LaMaze, F. (1970). *Painless Childbirth*. Chicago: Henry Regnery.

Langer, E. J., Janis, I. L., & Wolfer, J. A. "Reduction of Psychological Stress in Surgical Patients." *Journal Of Experimental Social Psychology*. 11, 155-165.

Langer, E. J., & Rodin, J. (1976). "The Effects of Choice and Enhanced Personal Responsibility for the Aged: A Field Experiment In an Institutional Setting." *Journal of Personality and Social Psychology*. 34 (2), 191-198.

Langer, E. J., & Rodin, J. (1977). "Long-Term Effects of a Control-Relevant Intervention with the Institutionalized Aged." *Journal of Personality and Social Psychology*. 35 (12), 897-902.

Lawson, N. C. (1976). *Depression After Spinal Cord Injury: A Multimeasure Longitudinal Study*. Unpublished doctoral dissertation, University of Houston, Houston, TX.

Leape, L. L. (1989). *Unnecessary Surgery*. Health Services Research. 24 (3), 351-407.

Lesar, T. S., Briceland, L. L., Delcoure, K, Parmalee, J. C., Masta-Gornic, V., & Pohl, H. (1990). "Medication Prescribing Errors in a Teaching Hospital." *Journal of the American Medical Association*. 263 (17), 2329-2334.

Leventhal, E. A., Leventhal, H. L., Shacham, S., & Easterling, D. V. (1989). "Active Coping Reduces Reports of Pain from Childbirth." *Journal of Consulting and Clinical Psychology*. 57 (3), 365-371.

Lia-Hoagberg, B., Rode, P., Bellfield, K., & Skovholt, C. (1988). *Barriers and Motivators to Prenatal Care: Experiences of Low-Income Women*. A Collaborative Community Study, Minneapolis, MN: Author.

Lieberman, M. A., Yalom, I. D., & Miles, M. B. (1973). *Encounter Groups: First Facts*. New York: Basic Books, Inc.

Long, J. W. (1992). *The Essential Guide to Prescription Drugs*. New York, N. Y., New York: Harper & Row.

Maerki, S. C., Luft, H. S., & Hunt, S. S. (1986). "Selecting Categories of Patients for Regionalization." *Medical Care*. 24

(2), 148-158.

Marks, I. (1971). "Phobic Disorders Four Years After Treatment: A Prospective Follow-Up." *British Journal of Psychiatry*. 118, 683-688.

McClure, W. (1985). "Buying Right: The Consequences of Glut." *Business and Health*. Vol. 2 (9), 43-46.

Mehling, A. (1985). *Recent Developments in Living Will Legislation and Other Significant Right-To-Die Gains*. News From Society for the Right to Die. June. (available from the society for the right to die, 250 west 57th street, New York, NY 10019.

Millenson, M. (1990). "Incentives on Trial." *Physician's Weekly*. June 4.

Melloni, J. B. (1985). *Melloni's Illustrated Medical Dictionary*. Williams & Wilkins.

Miller, S. M., Leinbach, A., & Brody, D. S. (1989). "Coping Style in Hypertensive Patients: Nature and Consequences." *Journal of Consulting and Clinical Psychology*. 57 (3), 333-337.

Minnesota, State of. (1989) *Patients and Residents of Health Care Facilities: Bill of Rights*. Minnesota Statutes Section 144.651.

Mooney, T., Cole, T., & Chilgren, R. (1975). *Sexual Options for Paraplegics and Quadriplegics*. Boston: Little, Brown & Co.

Nadel, C. & Portadin, G. (1977). "Sickle Cell Crises." *New York State Journal of Medicine*. June, 1075-1078.

New Good Housekeeping Family Health and Medical Guide. (1989) William Morrow and Company, Inc. New York, N.Y.

Orr, R. (1990, September). "Transforming the Hospital — A Response to a New View of a More Active Patient." In P. Drury (Chair), *Expanding Patients' Roles and Responsibilities: A New Dimension in Cost Management*. Presentation given at a meeting sponsored by the Minnesota Coalition on Health, Minneapolis, Minnesota.

Orynx Press, *Consumer Health & Nutrition Index*. (ISSN 0883-1963).

Peterson, C. & Seligman, M. E. P. (1987). "Explanatory Style and Illness." *Journal of Personality*, 55, 237-265.

Physician's Desk Reference. (1993). Oradell, N.J.: Medical Economics Company Inc.

Powell, L. H., Friedman, M., & Thoresen, C. (1984). "Can the Type A Behavior Pattern be Altered After Myocardial Infarction? A Second-Year Report from the Coronary Prevention Project." *Psychosomatic Medicine*. 46, 293-313.

Pratt, P., & Sarewitz, E. (1988). *General Surgery*. New York, N.Y.: Oxford.

Prior, A. (1987). "Personal View" *British Medical Journal*, 295, 920.

"Program Lowers Premature Birth Rate By 22 Percent." (1986, July). *Pulse*, 1-4.

Rahe, R. H., Ward, H. W., & Hayes, V. (1979). "Brief Group Therapy in Myocardial Infarction Rehabilitation: Three-to-Four-Year Follow-Up of a Controlled Trial." *Psychosomatic Medicine*. 41, 229-242.

Register, S. (1987). *Living With Chronic Illness. Days of Patience and Passion*. New York, NY: Macmillan.

Reiser, S. J. (1978). *Medicine and the Reign of Technology*. Cambridge: Cambridge University Press.

Rice, J. (1989). Personal communication.

Rich, E. C., Gifford, G., Luxenberg, M., & Dowd, B. (1990). "The Relationship of House Staff Experience to the Cost and Quality of Inpatient Care." *Journal of the American Medical Association*. 263 (7), 953- 957.

Rosenman, R. H., Brand, R. J. et al. (1975). "Coronary Heart Disease in the Western Collaborative Group Study: Final Follow-Up of Eight and One-Half Years." *Journal of the American Medical Association*. 233, 872-877.

Schaller, W. E., & Carroll, C R. (1976) *Health, Quackery and the Consumer*. Philadelphia: W. B. Saunders.

Schleifer, S. J., Keller, S. E., Camerino, M., Thornton, J. C., & Stein, M. (1983). "Suppression of Lymphocyte Stimulation Following Bereavement." *Journal of the American Medical Association*. 250 (3), 374-377.

Schoener, G. R., Milgrom, J. H., Gonsiorek, J. C., Luepker, E. T., Conroe, R. M. (1989). *Psychotherapists' Sexual Involvement with Clients*. Minneapolis: Walk-In Counseling Center

Schover, L. R., & Jensen, S. B. (1988). *Sexuality and Chronic*

Illness. New York: The Guilford Press.

Schuman, D. M. (1990). "Point/Counterpoint." *Physician's Weekly*. 7 (24).

Seligman, M. E. P., & Maier, S. F. (1967). "Failure to Escape Traumatic Shock." *Journal of Experimental Psychology*. 74 (1), 1-9.

Siegel, B. (1986). *Love, Medicine, & Miracles*. New York, NY: Harper & Row.

Simonton, C., & Simonton, S. (1978). *Getting Well Again: A Step-by-Step Self-Help Guide to Overcoming Cancer for Patients and Their Families*. Los Angeles, CA: J. P. Tarcher.

Slack, W. V. (1972). "Patient Power: A Patient-Oriented Value System." In John Jacquez (Ed.), *Proceedings of the Second Conference on the Diagnostic Process held at the University of Michigan* (pp. 3-7). Charles C. Thomas: Publisher.

Slack, W. V. (1977). "The Patient's Right to Decide." *Lancet*, July, 240.

Sneddon, J. (1980). "Myasthenia Gravis: A Study of Social, Medical, and Emotional Problems In 26 Patients." *Lancet*. 1, 526.

Spiegel, D., Bloom, J. R., Kraemer, H. C., & Gottheil, E. (1989). "Effect of Psychosocial Treatment on Survival of Patients with Metastatic Breast Cancer." *Lancet*. October, 888-891.

Spooner, R. F. (1987). "Crohn's Disease." In H. Mandell & H.
Spiro (Eds.), *When Doctors Get Sick* (pp. 229-241). New York and London: Plenum. [fictitious name]

Strauss, D. H., Spitzer, R. L., & Muskin, P. R. (1990). "Maladaptive Denial of Physical Illness: A Proposal for DSM-IV." *The American Journal of Psychiatry*. 147, 1168-1172.

Suls, J. & Wan, C. K. (1989). "Effects of Sensory and Procedural Information on Coping with Stressful Medical Procedures and Pain: A Meta-Analysis." *Journal of Consulting and Clinical Psychology*. 57 (3), 372-379.

The Wizard of OZ (1939). Noel Langley, Florence Ryerson, and Edgar Allan Woolf, screenplay; Metro-Goldwyn-Mayer.

Thomas, R. & Holbrook, T. (1987). "Sickle Cell Disease: Ways To Reduce Morbidity and Mortality." *Postgraduate Medi-*

cine, 81 (5), 265-280.

Ulrich, R. S. (1983). "View Through a Window May Influence Recovery from Surgery." *Science*. 224, 420-421.

Vernick, D. M. (1986). "Stapedectomy Results in a Residency Training Program." *Annals of Otology, Rhinology, and Laryngology*. 95, 477-479.

Visintainer, M. & Seligman, M. (1983). "The Hope Factor." *American Health*, July/August.

Wolinsky, F. D. (1988) *The Sociology Of Health*. (2nd ed.). Belmont, CA: Wadsworth Publishing Company.

Woolfolk, R. L. (1978). *Stress, Sanity, & Survival*. New York, N.Y.: Signet.

World Health Organization. (1958) *The World Health Organization: A Report on the First Ten Years*. Geneva, Switzerland: Author.

Wortman, C. B. & Silver, R. C. (1989). "The Myths of Coping with Loss." *Journal of Consulting and Clinical Psychology*. 57 (3), 349-357.

Yalom, I. D., & Leiberman, M. A. (1971d) "A Study of Encounter Group Casualties." *Archives of General Psychiatry*, 25D, 16-30.

Zako, L. (1989) "Point/Counterpoint." *Physician's Weekly*. Vol. VI, No. 14.